DICTIONARY OF KINETOGRAPHY LABAN
(LABANOTATION)

DICTIONARY OF KINETOGRAPHY LABAN

(Labanotation)

Albrecht Knust

Designed and drafted by
Diana Baddeley-Lange

Advisory assistance
Roderyk Lange

Illustrations by
Annemie Schoenfeldt-Juris

VOLUME II: EXAMPLES

MACDONALD AND EVANS

MACDONALD AND EVANS LTD.
Estover, Plymouth PL6 7PZ

First published 1979

©
MACDONALD AND EVANS LIMITED
1979

ISBN 0 7121 0416 X

Filmset and printed in Great Britain by
BAS Printers Limited, Over Wallop, Hampshire

Alphabet of Kinetography
Das Alphabet der Kinetographie
L'alphabet de la Cinétographie

The Four Principles

Die vier Grundsätze

Les Quatre Règles Fondamentales

right	right forward	turn to the right
rechts	rechtsvor	Wendung über rechts
à droite	en avant - à droite	tour vers la droite
1	2	3

high	medium level	low
hoch	mittelhoch	tief
haut	niveau moyen	bas
4 a	4 b	4 c

action stroke	passive or resulting movement	
Aktionsstrich	passive oder resultierende Bewegung	
trait d'action	mouvement passive ou résultant	
5 a	5 b	

successively
nacheinander
successivement

6 a

at the same time

gleichzeitig

simultanément

6 b

7

A

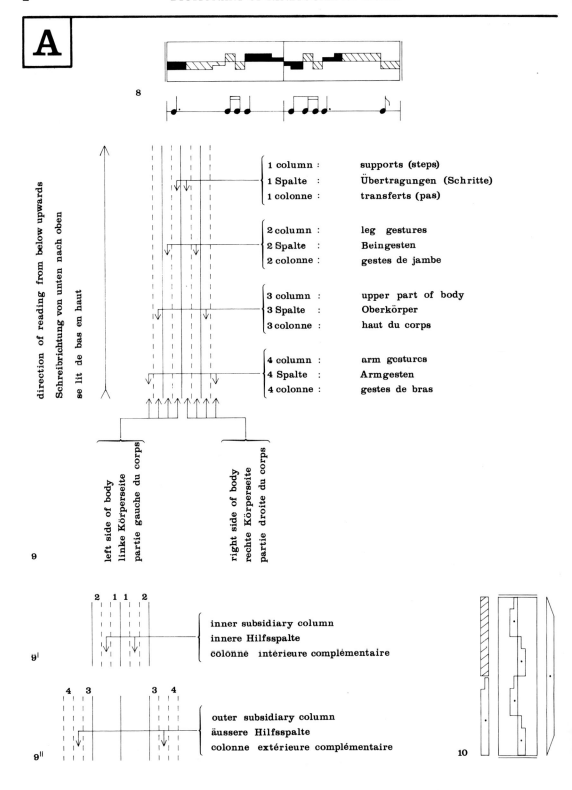

8

direction of reading from below upwards

Schreibrichtung von unten nach oben

se lit de bas en haut

1 column :	supports (steps)
1 Spalte :	Übertragungen (Schritte)
1 colonne :	transferts (pas)

2 column :	leg gestures
2 Spalte :	Beingesten
2 colonne :	gestes de jambe

3 column :	upper part of body
3 Spalte :	Oberkörper
3 colonne :	haut du corps

4 column :	arm gestures
4 Spalte :	Armgesten
4 colonne :	gestes de bras

left side of body
linke Körperseite
partie gauche du corps

right side of body
rechte Körperseite
partie droite du corps

9

2 1 1 2

inner subsidiary column
innere Hilfsspalte
colonne intérieure complémentaire

9ᴵ

4 3   3 4

outer subsidiary column
äussere Hilfsspalte
colonne extérieure complémentaire

9ᴵᴵ

10

A

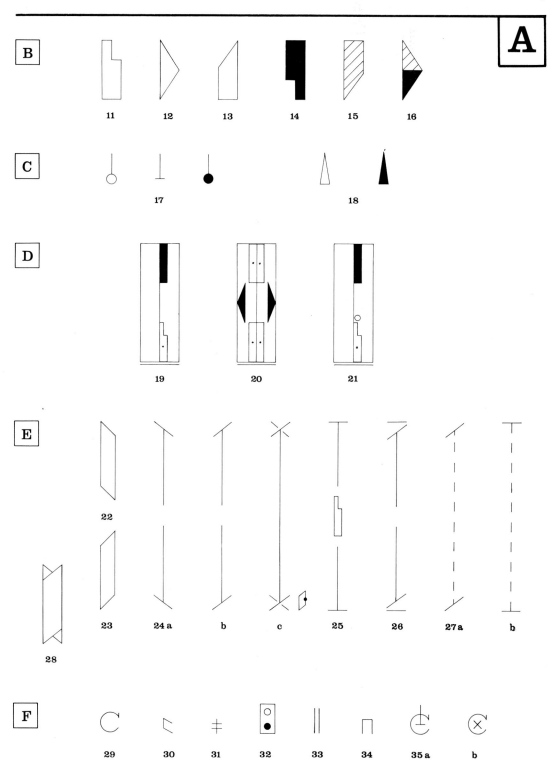

B 11 12 13 14 15 16

C 17 18

D 19 20 21

E 22 23 24a b c 25 26 27a b 28

F 29 30 31 32 33 34 35a b

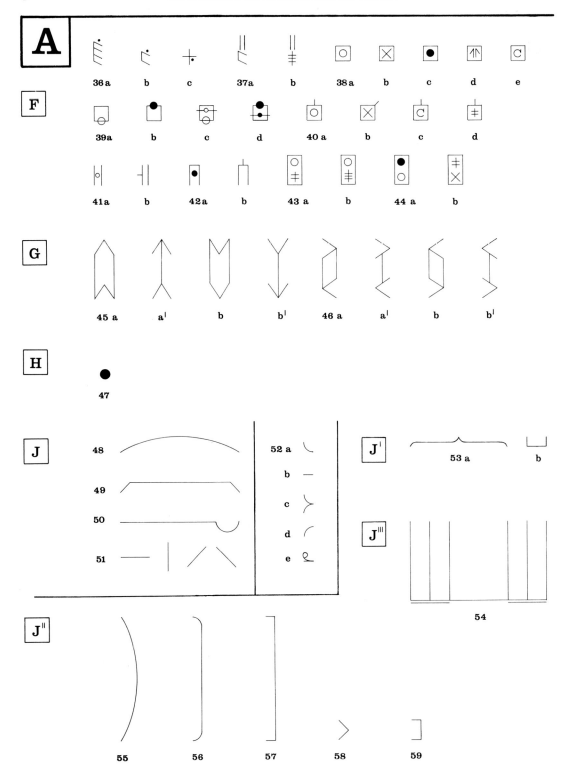

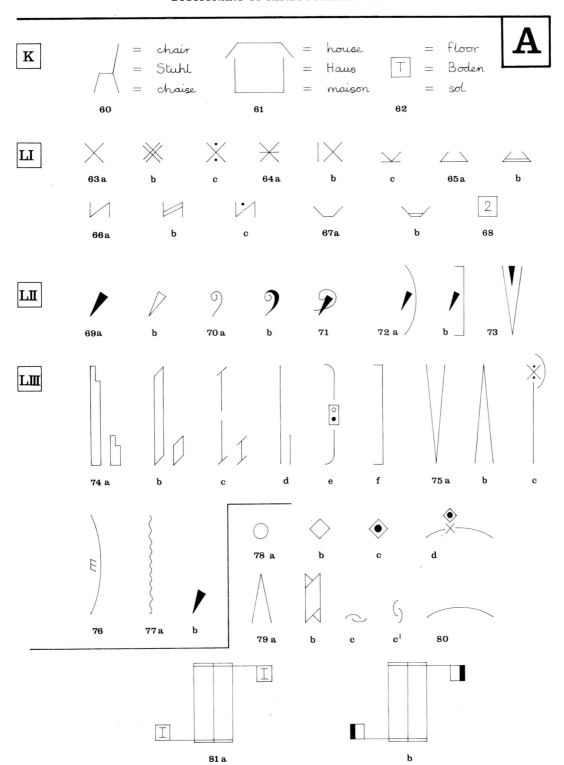

K 60 = chair / Stuhl / chaise
61 = house / Haus / maison
62 = floor / Boden / sol

A

LI 63a b c 64a b c 65a b
66a b c 67a b 68

LII 69a b 70a b 71 72a b 73

LIII 74a b c d e f 75a b c
76 77a b 78a b c d 79a b c c' 80
81a b

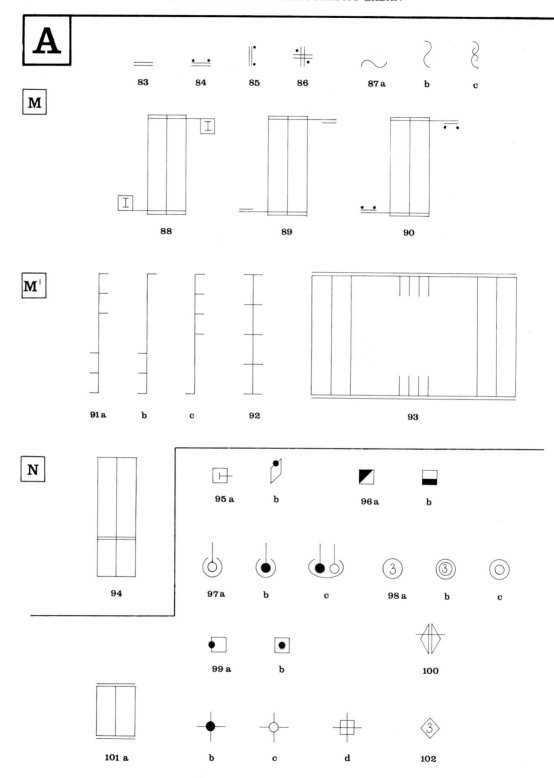

Direction Signs
Die Richtungszeichen
Les signes de direction

F	=	forward	V	=	vor	Av	=	en avant
B	=	backward	Z	=	zurück	Arr	=	en arrière
R	=	to the right	R	=	rechts	Dr	=	à droite
L	=	to the left	L	=	links	G	=	à gauche
H	=	high	H	=	hoch	H	=	en haut
D	=	deep	T	=	tief	B	=	en bas
Pl	=	in place	Pl	=	am Platz	Pl	=	en place

103

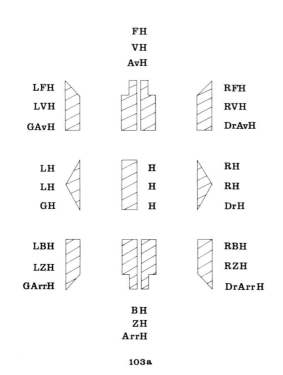

103a

B

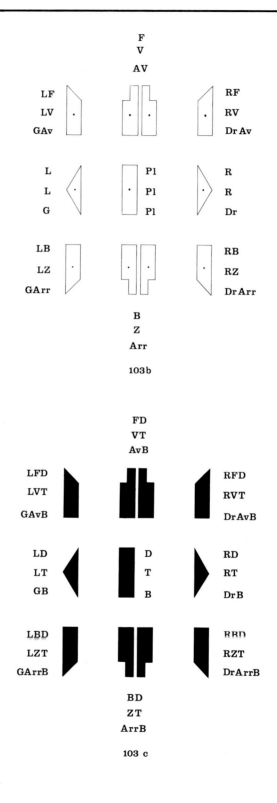

F
V
AV

LF		RF
LV		RV
GAv		Dr Av

L	Pl	R
L	Pl	R
G	Pl	Dr

LB		RB
LZ		RZ
GArr		Dr Arr

B
Z
Arr

103b

FD
VT
AvB

LFD		RFD
LVT		RVT
GAvB		DrAvB

LD	D	RD
LT	T	RT
GB	B	DrB

LBD		RBD
LZT		RZT
GArrB		DrArrB

BD
ZT
ArrB

103 c

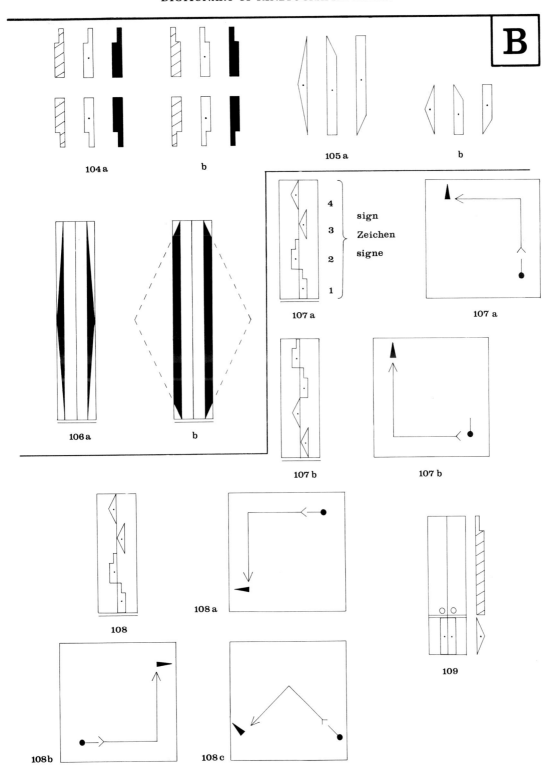

104 a   b   105 a   b

sign
Zeichen
signe

106 a   b   107 a   107 a

107 b   107 b

108   108 a   109

108 b   108 c

B

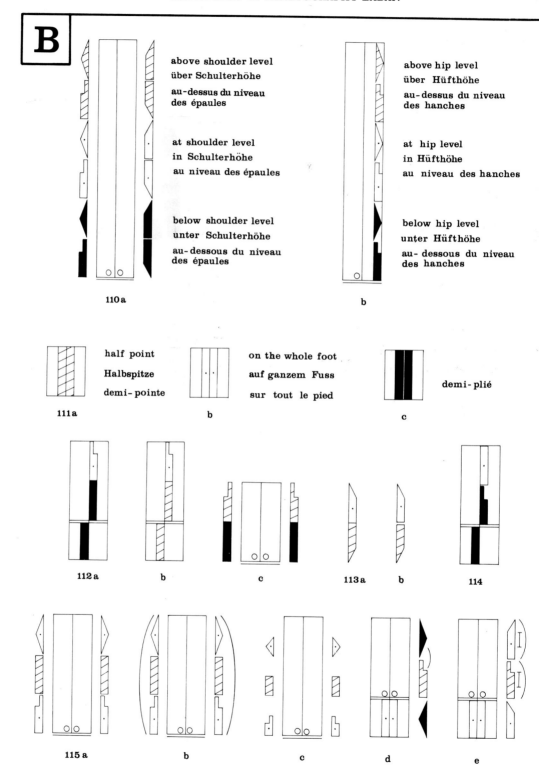

above shoulder level
über Schulterhöhe
au-dessus du niveau
des épaules

at shoulder level
in Schulterhöhe
au niveau des épaules

below shoulder level
unter Schulterhöhe
au-dessous du niveau
des épaules

110 a

above hip level
über Hüfthöhe
au-dessus du niveau
des hanches

at hip level
in Hüfthöhe
au niveau des hanches

below hip level
unter Hüfthöhe
au-dessous du niveau
des hanches

b

half point
Halbspitze
demi-pointe

111 a

on the whole foot
auf ganzem Fuss
sur tout le pied

b

demi-plié

c

112 a   b   c   113 a   b   114

115 a   b   c   d   e

B

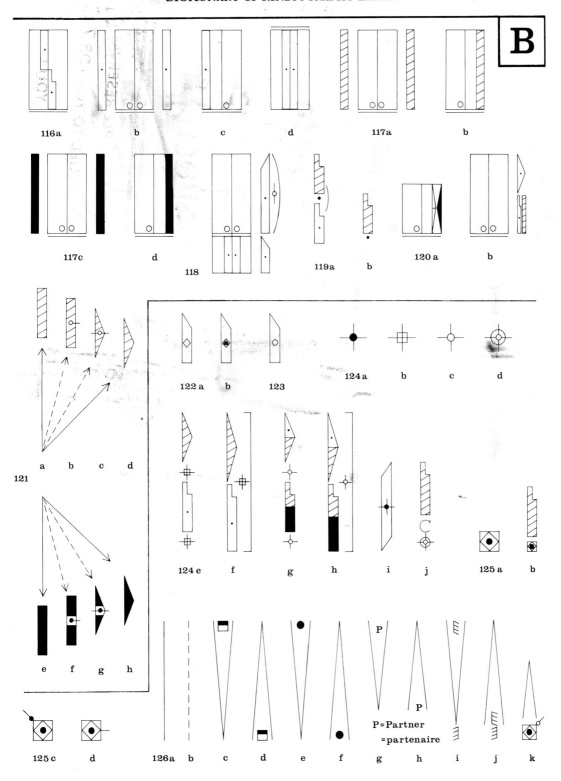

116a   b   c   d   117a   b

117c   d   118   119a   b   120 a   b

121
a   b   c   d

e   f   g   h

122 a   b   123   124a   b   c   d

124 e   f   g   h   i   j   125 a   b

P

P

P=Partner
=partenaire

125 c   d   126a   b   c   d   e   f   g   h   i   j   k

C Pin Signs
Die Positionszeichen
Les signes de position

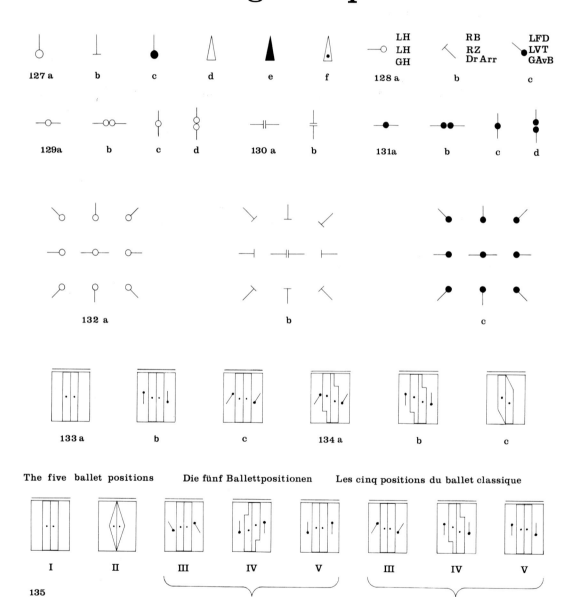

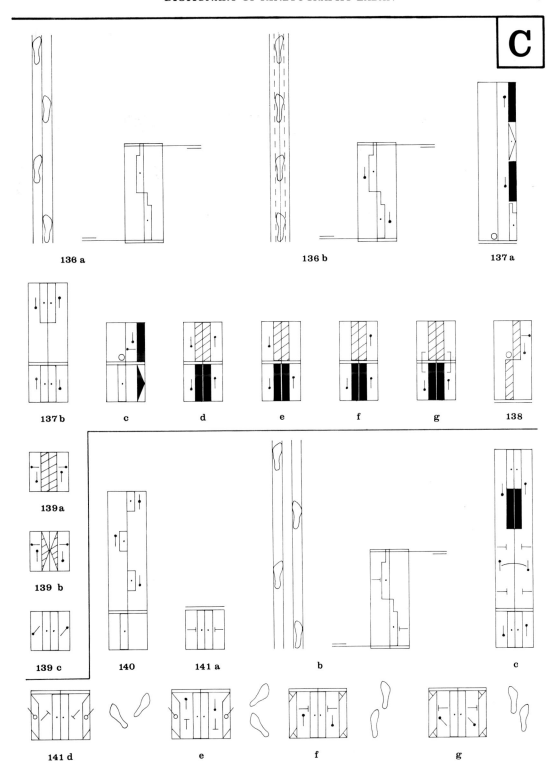

C

136 a

136 b

137 a

137 b

c

d

e

f

g

138

139 a

139 b

139 c

140

141 a

b

c

141 d

e

f

g

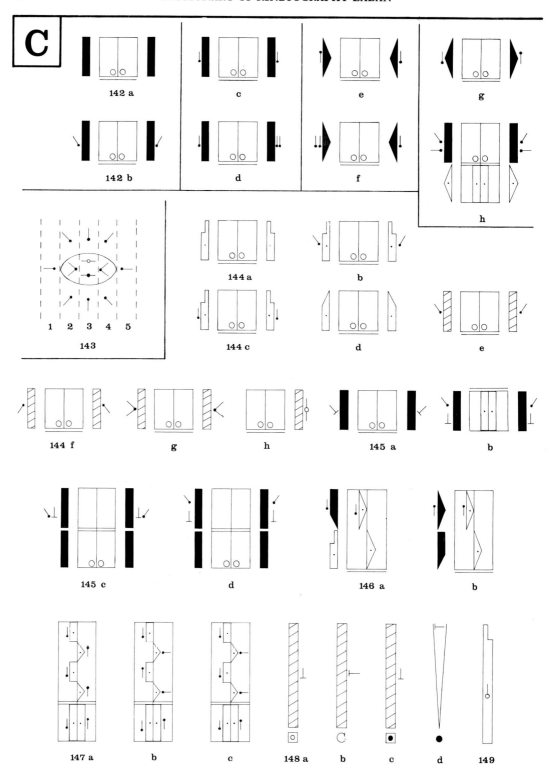

142 a

c

e

g

142 b

d

f

h

143

1   2   3   4   5

144 a

b

144 c

d

e

144 f

g

h

145 a

b

145 c

d

146 a

b

147 a

b

c

148 a

b

c

d

149

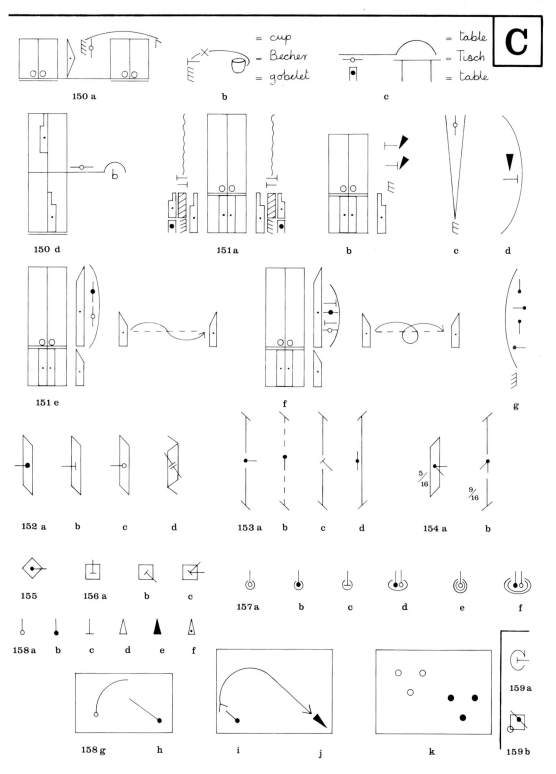

= cup
= Becher
= gobelet

= table
= Tisch
= table

150 a   b   c

150 d   151 a   b   c   d

151 e   f   g

152 a   b   c   d   153 a   b   c   d   154 a   b

155   156 a   b   c   157 a   b   c   d   e   f

158 a   b   c   d   e   f

158 g   h   i   j   k   159 a

159 b

Supports
Die Übertragungen
Les transferts

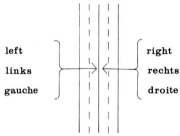

left   right
links   rechts
gauche   droite

160

support column

Übertragungsspalte

colonnes de transferts

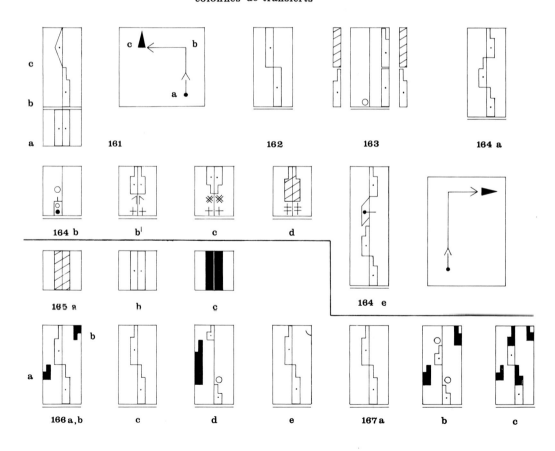

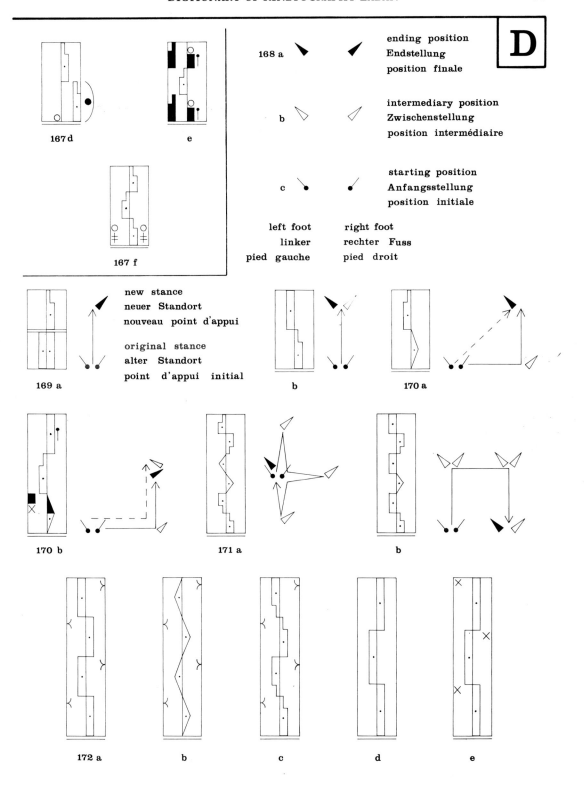

D

167 d

e

167 f

168 a — ending position
Endstellung
position finale

b — intermediary position
Zwischenstellung
position intermédiaire

c — starting position
Anfangsstellung
position initiale

left foot — right foot
linker — rechter Fuss
pied gauche — pied droit

new stance
neuer Standort
nouveau point d'appui

original stance
alter Standort
point d'appui initial

169 a

b

170 a

170 b

171 a

b

172 a

b

c

d

e

D

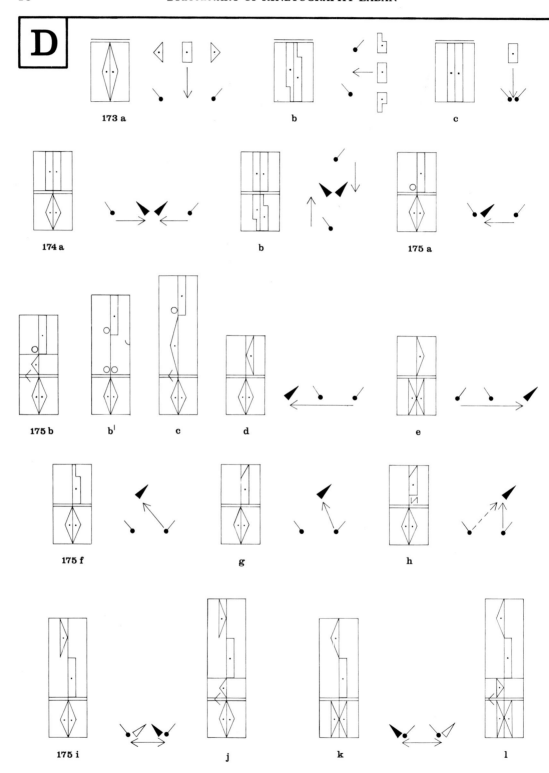

173 a   b   c

174 a   b   175 a

175 b   b'   c   d   e

175 f   g   h

175 i   j   k   l

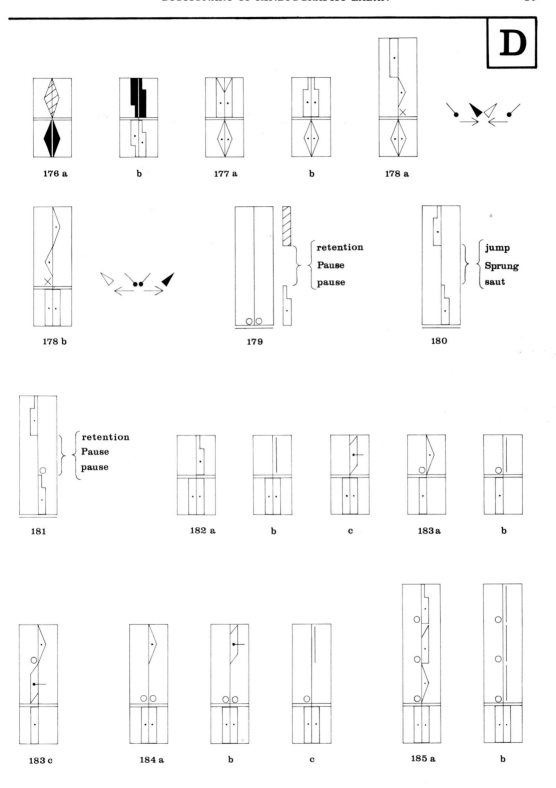

D

176 a   b   177 a   b   178 a

178 b   179   {retention / Pause / pause}   180   {jump / Sprung / saut}

181   {retention / Pause / pause}   182 a   b   c   183 a   b

183 c   184 a   b   c   185 a   b

D

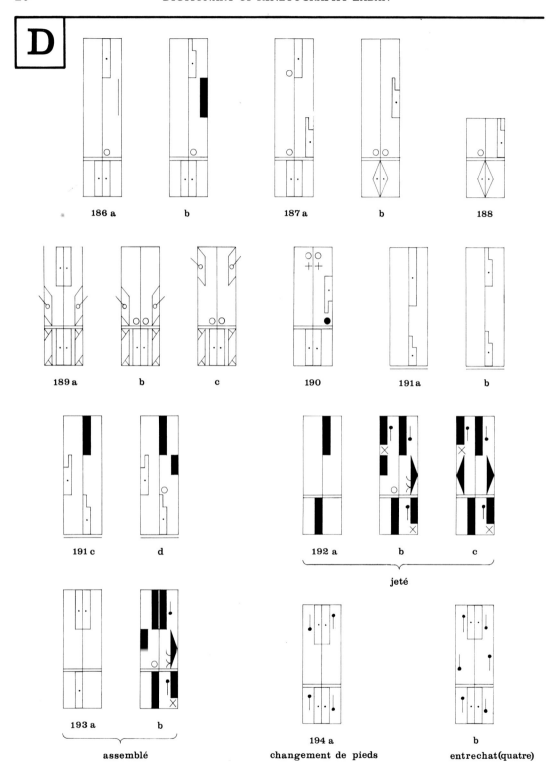

186 a   b   187 a   b   188

189 a   b   c   190   191 a   b

191 c   d   192 a   b   c

jeté

193 a   b

assemblé

194 a
changement de pieds

b
entrechat (quatre)

D

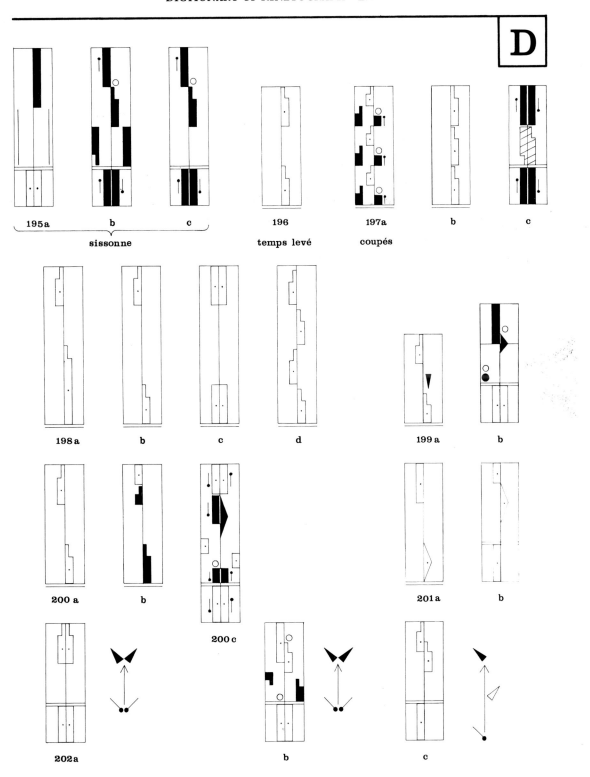

195a   b   c

sissonne   temps levé   coupés

196   197a   b   c

198 a   b   c   d   199 a   b

200 a   b   201a   b

200 c

202a   b   c

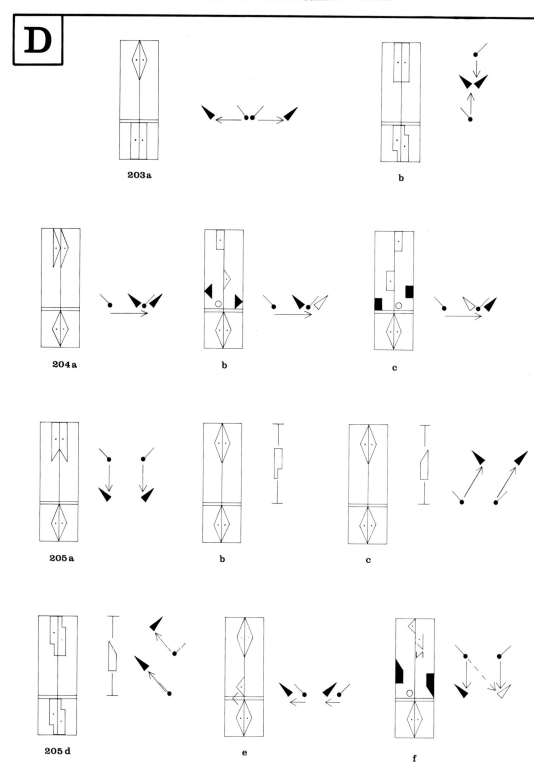

D

203a   b

204a   b   c

205a   b   c

205d   e   f

D

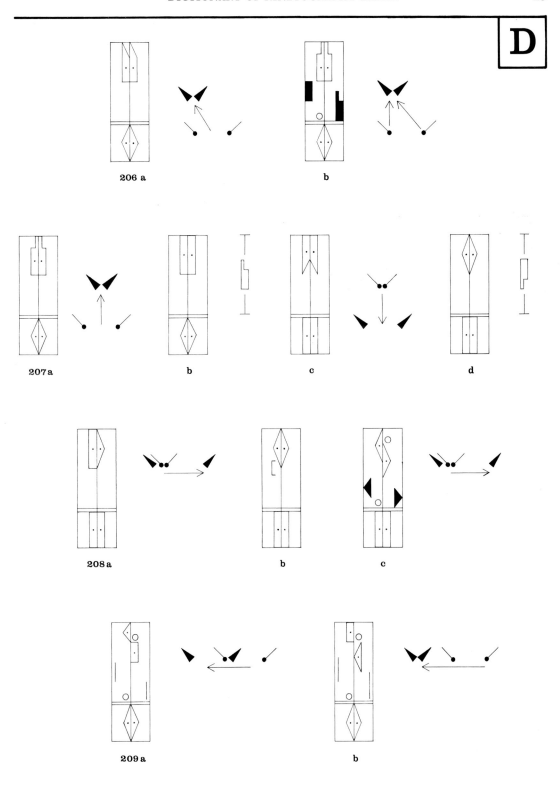

206 a   b

207 a   b   c   d

208 a   b   c

209 a   b

D

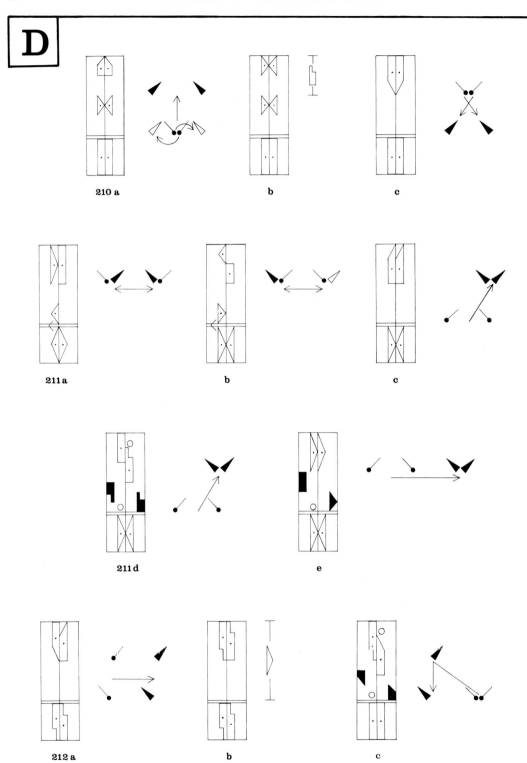

210 a   b   c

211 a   b   c

211 d   e

212 a   b   c

D

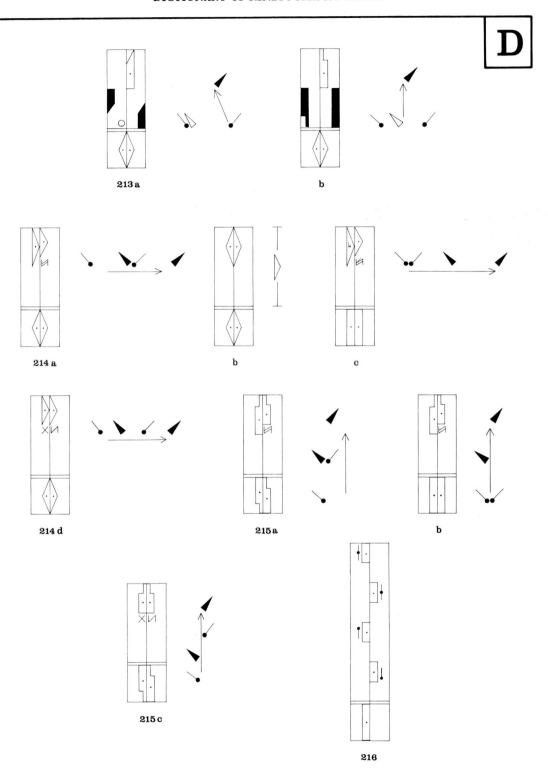

213 a   b

214 a   b   c

214 d   215 a   b

215 c

216

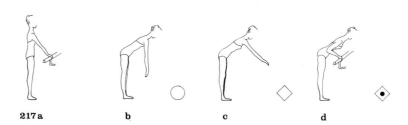

217a   b   c   d

<table>
e Retention in the body
Pause im Körper
Pause dans le corps

f   Retention in space
Pause im Raum
Pause dans l'espace
</table>

Retention in the body
Pause im Körper
Pause dans le corps

Retention in space
Pause im Raum
Pause dans l'espace

g   **Retention on a spot**
Pause am Ort
Pause au lieu

h

i   **Standard retention**
Standardpause
Pause standard

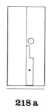 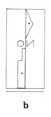 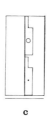 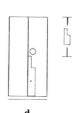 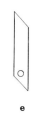

218a   b   c   d   e

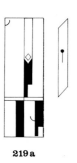

219a

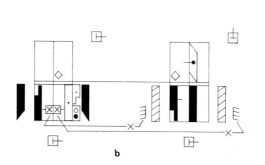

b

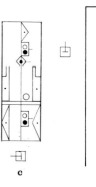

c

P ◇
219d

P
◇
219e

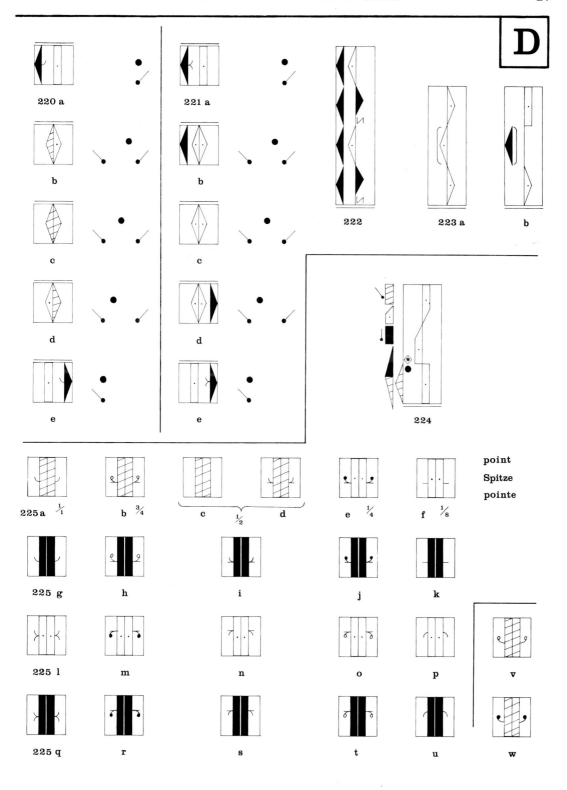

D

220 a

b

c

d

e

221 a

b

c

d

e

222

223 a

b

224

225 a $\frac{1}{1}$ b $\frac{3}{4}$ c $\frac{1}{2}$ d   e $\frac{1}{4}$ f $\frac{1}{8}$

point
Spitze
pointe

225 g   h   i   j   k

225 l   m   n   o   p   v

225 q   r   s   t   u   w

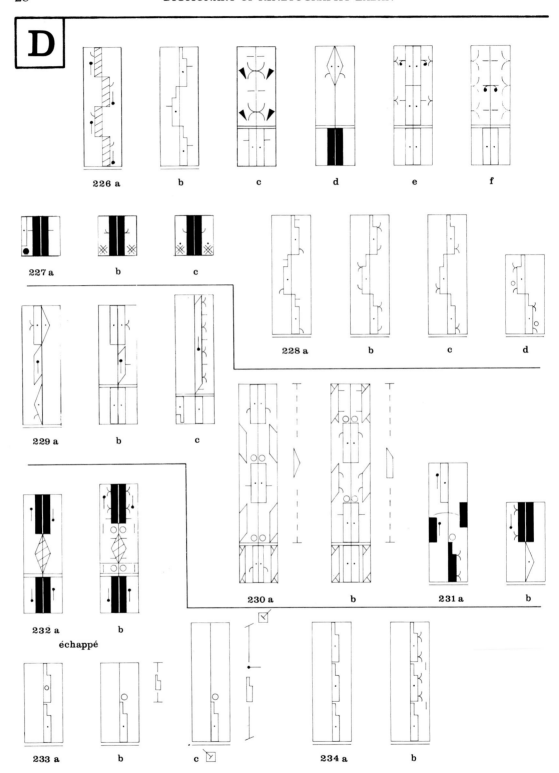

226 a   b   c   d   e   f

227 a   b   c   228 a   b   c   d

229 a   b   c

230 a   b   231 a   b

232 a   b
échappé

233 a   b   c   234 a   b

Floor Patterns
Der Bodenweg
Le tracé du parcours

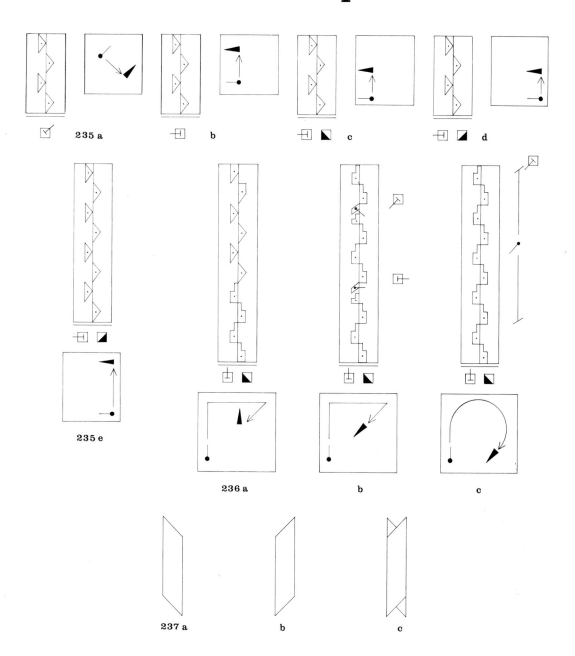

235 a   b   c   d

235 e

236 a   b   c

237 a   b   c

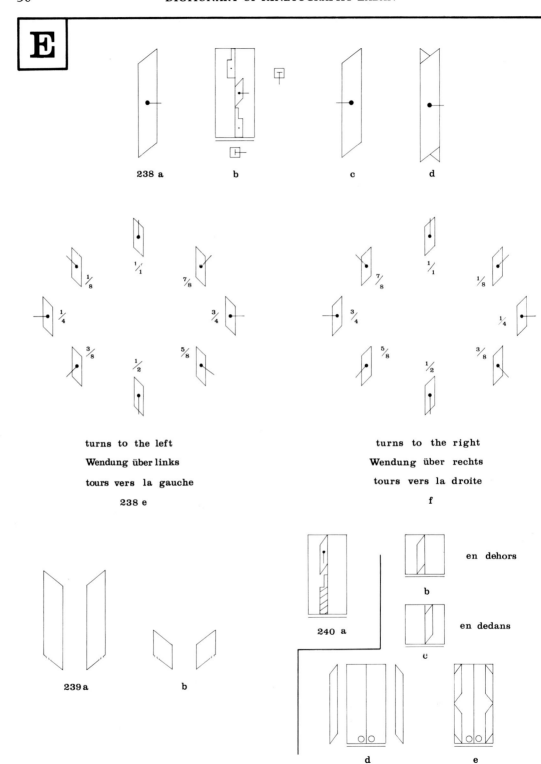

238 a   b   c   d

turns to the left
Wendung über links
tours vers la gauche
238 e

turns to the right
Wendung über rechts
tours vers la droite
f

239 a   b

240 a

en dehors
b

en dedans
c

d   e

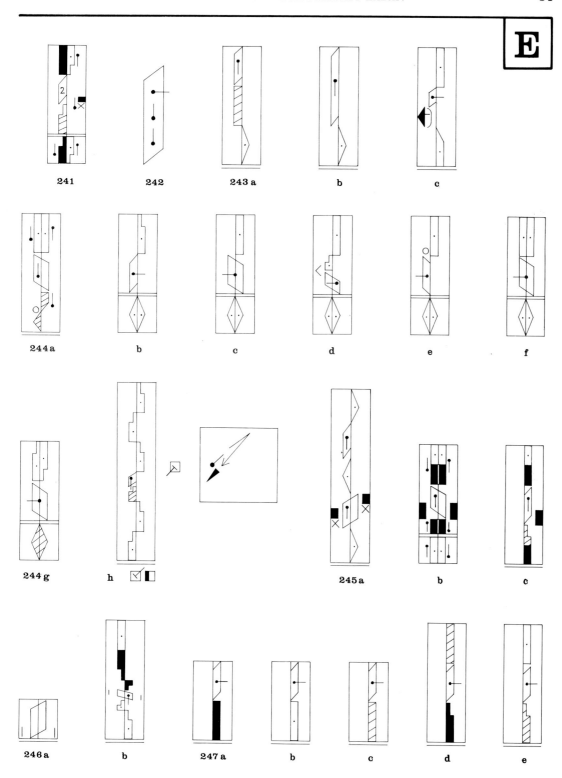

241   242   243 a   b   c

244 a   b   c   d   e   f

244 g   h   245 a   b   c

246 a   b   247 a   b   c   d   e

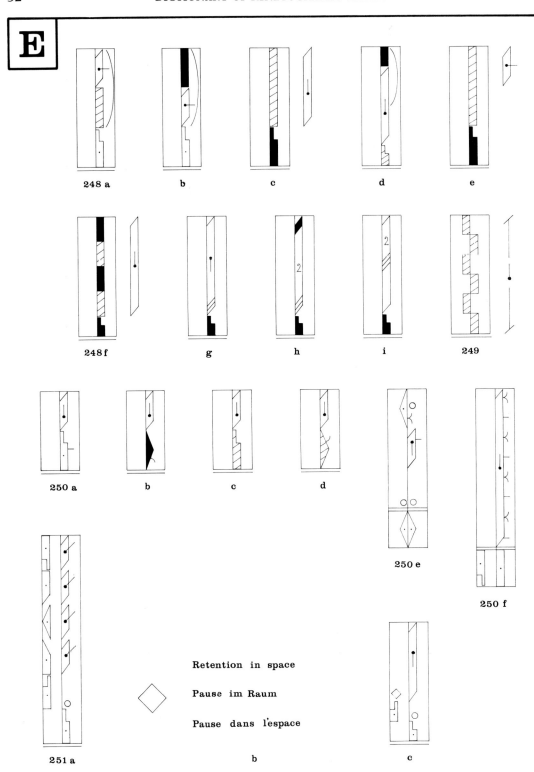

248 a

b

c

d

e

248 f

g

h

i

249

250 a

b

c

d

250 e

250 f

Retention in space

Pause im Raum

Pause dans l'espace

251 a

b

c

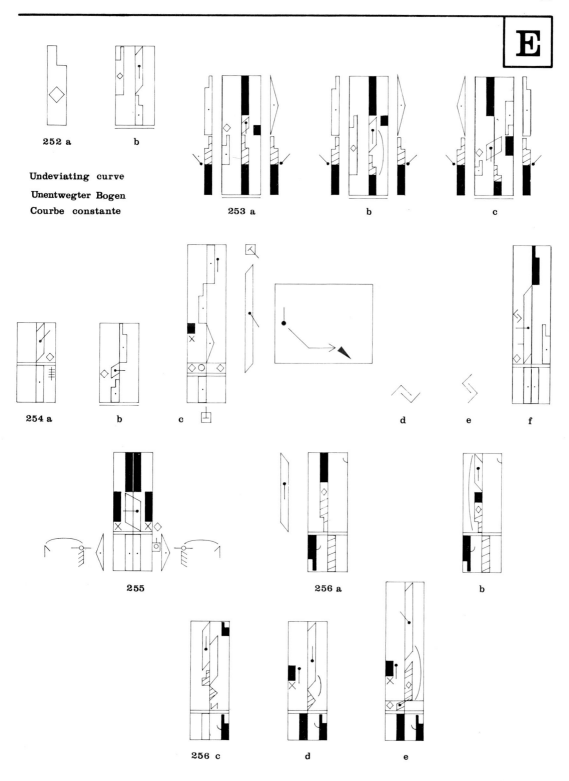

E

252 a   b

Undeviating curve
Unentwegter Bogen
Courbe constante

253 a   b   c

254 a   b   c   d   e   f

255   256 a   b

256 c   d   e

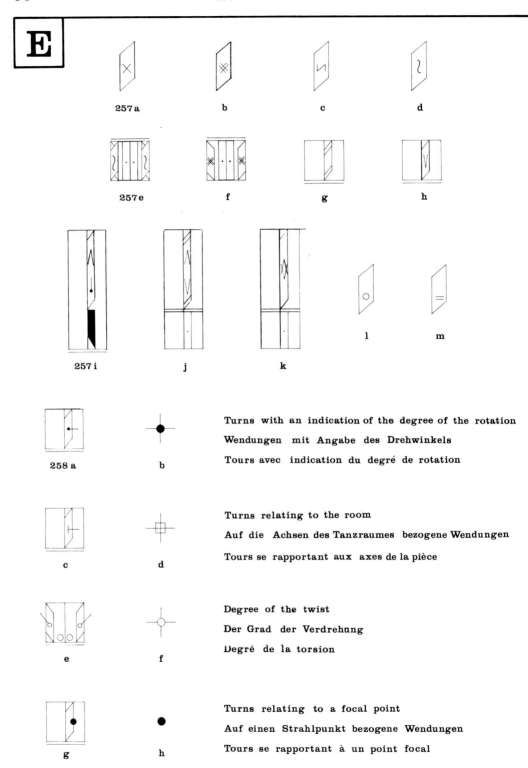

257 a   b   c   d

257 e   f   g   h

257 i   j   k   l   m

258 a   b

Turns with an indication of the degree of the rotation

Wendungen mit Angabe des Drehwinkels

Tours avec indication du degré de rotation

c   d

Turns relating to the room

Auf die Achsen des Tanzraumes bezogene Wendungen

Tours se rapportant aux axes de la pièce

e   f

Degree of the twist

Der Grad der Verdrehung

Degré de la torsion

g   h

Turns relating to a focal point

Auf einen Strahlpunkt bezogene Wendungen

Tours se rapportant à un point focal

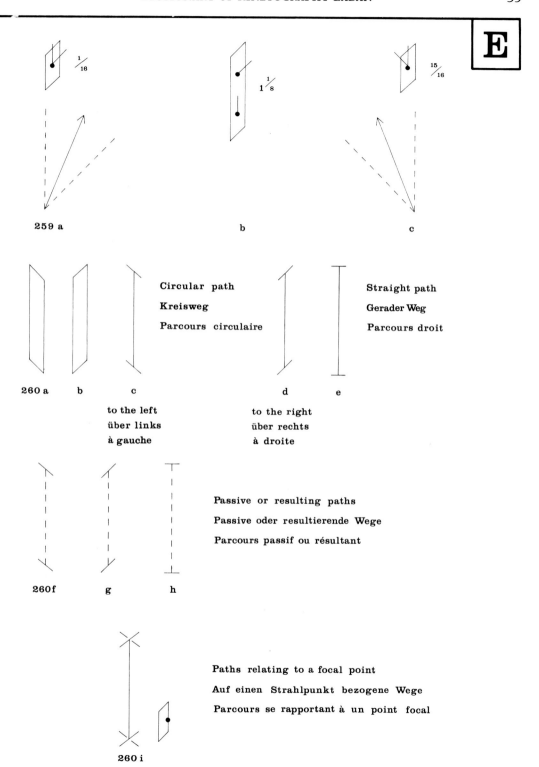

259 a

b

c

Circular path
Kreisweg
Parcours circulaire

Straight path
Gerader Weg
Parcours droit

260 a   b   c   d   e

to the left
über links
à gauche

to the right
über rechts
à droite

Passive or resulting paths
Passive oder resultierende Wege
Parcours passif ou résultant

260 f   g   h

Paths relating to a focal point
Auf einen Strahlpunkt bezogene Wege
Parcours se rapportant à un point focal

260 i

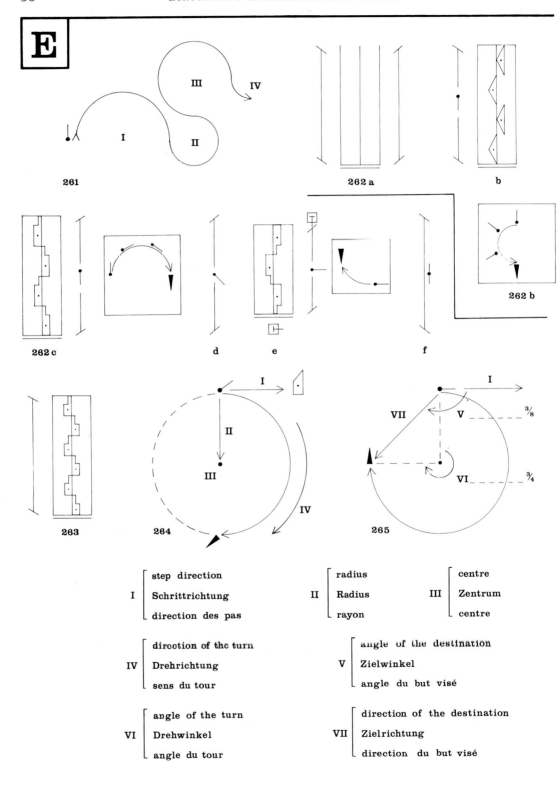

261   262 a   b

262 c   d   e   f   262 b

263   264   265

I	step direction	II	radius	III	centre
	Schrittrichtung		Radius		Zentrum
	direction des pas		rayon		centre

IV	direction of the turn	V	angle of the destination
	Drehrichtung		Zielwinkel
	sens du tour		angle du but visé

VI	angle of the turn	VII	direction of the destination
	Drehwinkel		Zielrichtung
	angle du tour		direction du but visé

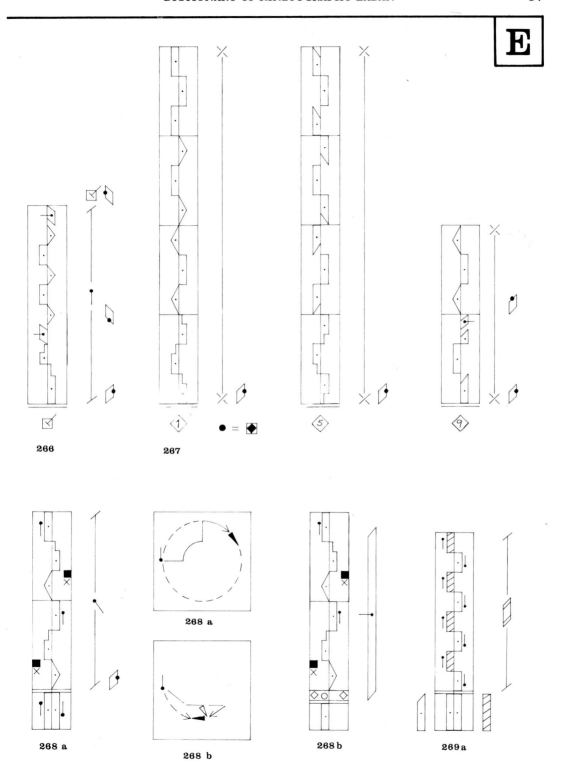

266

267

● = ◆

268 a

268 a

268 b

268 b

269a

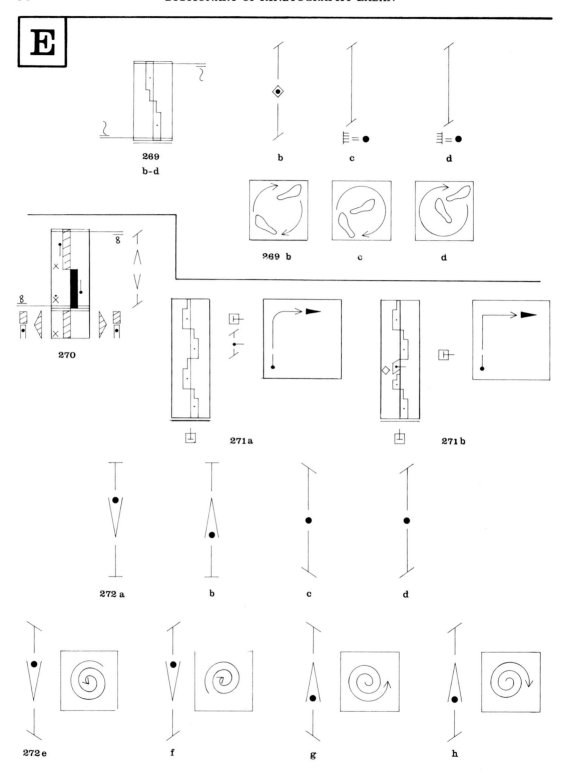

269
b-d

b

c

d

269 b

c

d

270

271a

271b

272 a

b

c

d

272 e

f

g

h

E

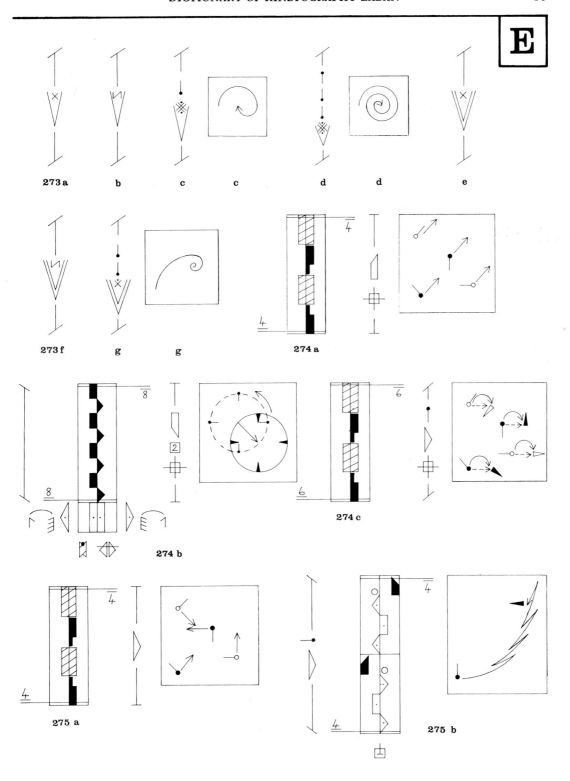

273 a   b   c   c   d   d   e

273 f   g   g   274 a

274 b   274 c

275 a   275 b

E

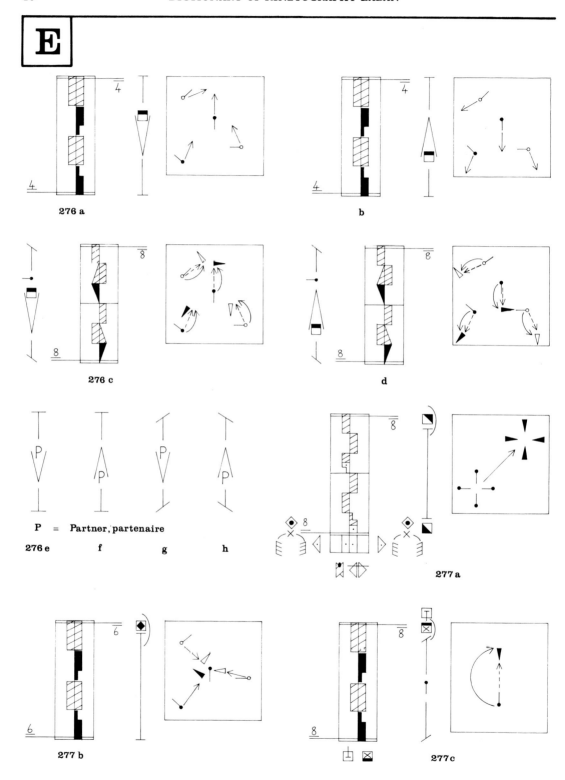

276 a

b

276 c

d

P = Partner, partenaire

276 e   f   g   h

277 a

277 b

277 c

E

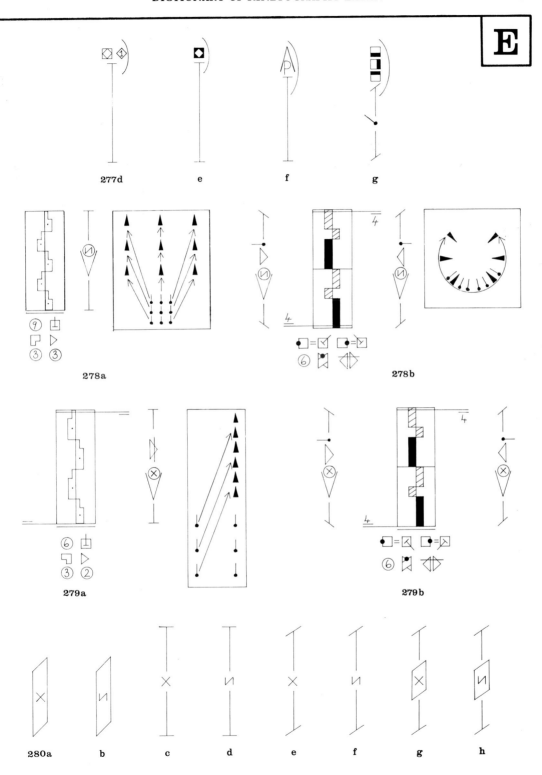

277d   e   f   g

278a   278b

279a   279b

280a   b   c   d   e   f   g   h

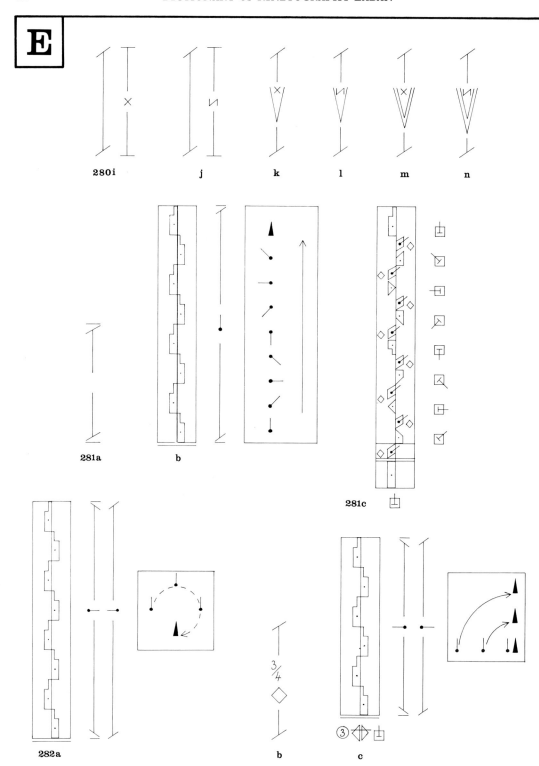

280i   j   k   l   m   n

281a   b

281c

282a   b   c

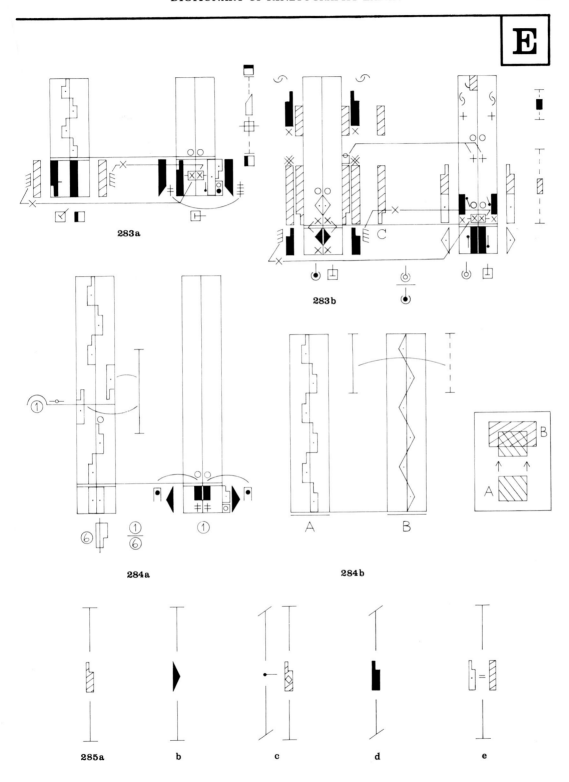

283a

283b

284a

284b

285a   b   c   d   e

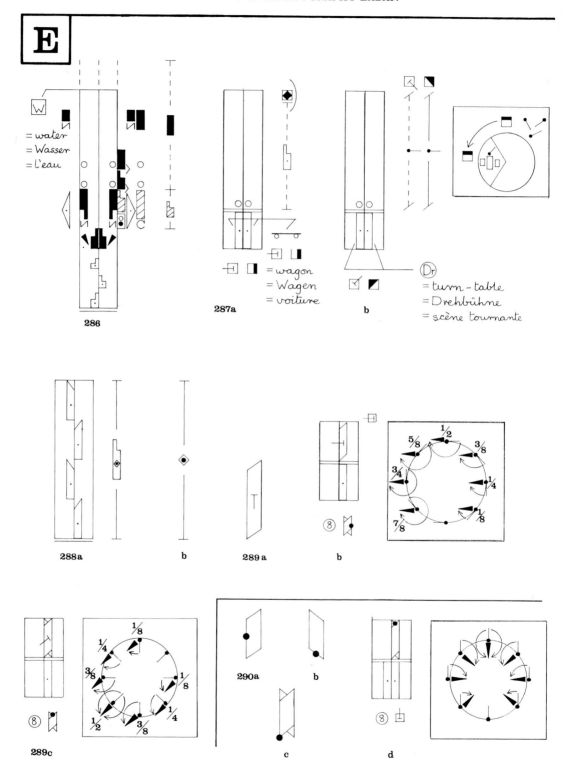

E

= water
= Wasser
= l'eau

286

287a
= wagon
= Wagen
= voiture

b
= turn – table
= Drehbühne
= scène tournante

288a   **b**   **289 a**   **b**

289c

290a   **b**

c   **d**

E

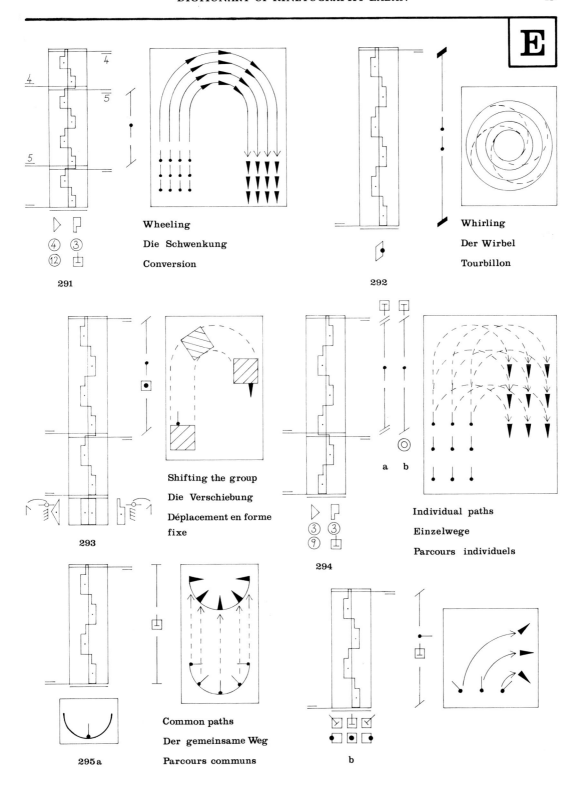

Wheeling

Die Schwenkung

Conversion

291

Whirling

Der Wirbel

Tourbillon

292

Shifting the group

Die Verschiebung

Déplacement en forme fixe

293

Individual paths

Einzelwege

Parcours individuels

a   b

294

Common paths

Der gemeinsame Weg

Parcours communs

295a

b

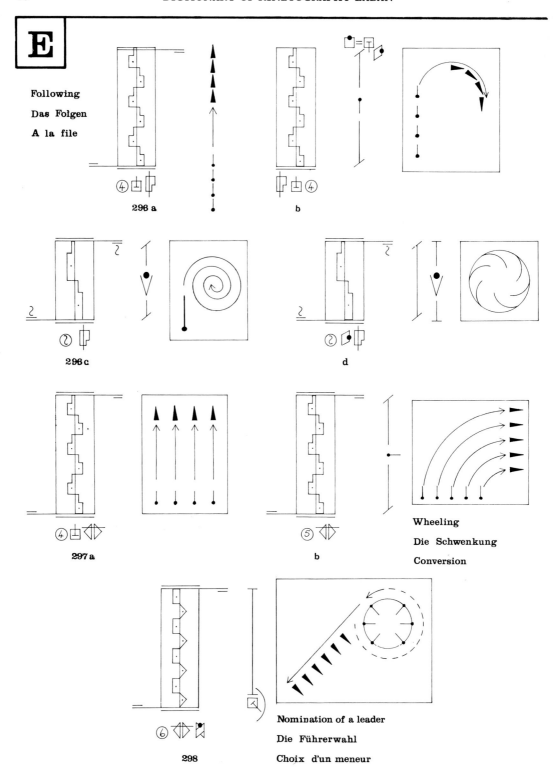

E

Following

Das Folgen

A la file

296 a

b

296 c

d

297 a

b

Wheeling

Die Schwenkung

Conversion

298

Nomination of a leader

Die Führerwahl

Choix d'un meneur

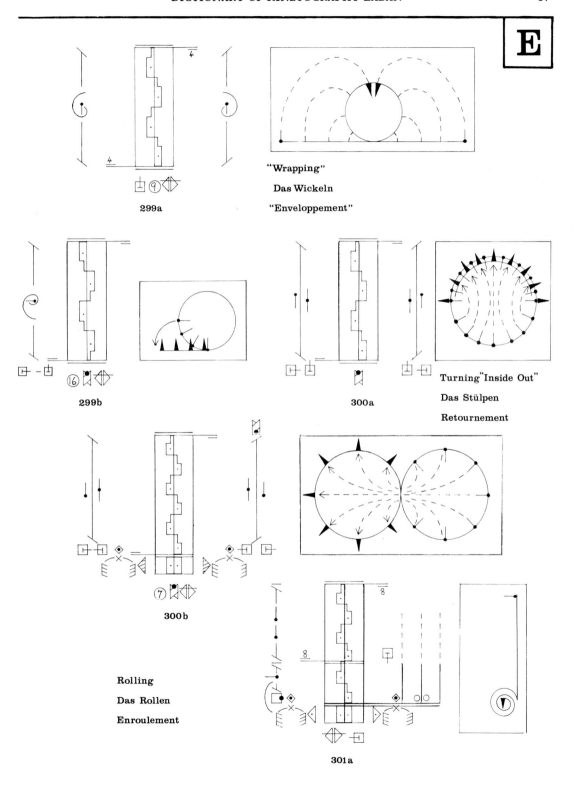

E

"Wrapping"

Das Wickeln

"Enveloppement"

299a

299b

300a

Turning "Inside Out"

Das Stülpen

Retournement

300b

Rolling

Das Rollen

Enroulement

301a

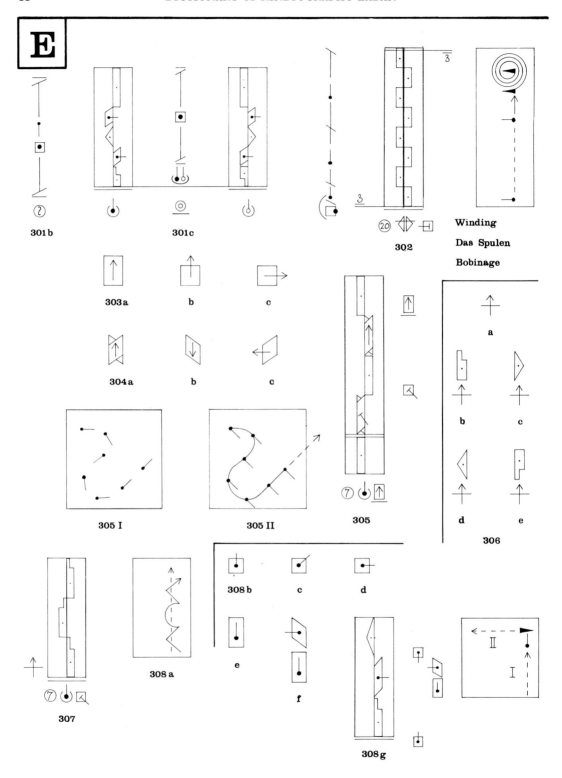

E

301 b

301 c

302

Winding

Das Spulen

Bobinage

303 a   b   c

304 a   b   c

305 I   305 II   305

306

a

b   c

d   e

307

308 a

308 b   c   d

e

f

308 g

E

309

310 = starting front
= Anfangsfront
= front de départ

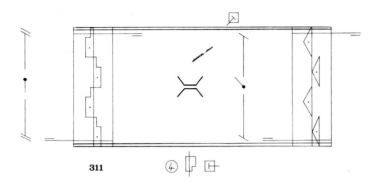

311

311 I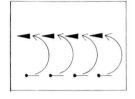

II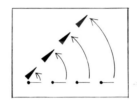

III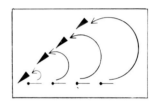

312a b c d e f

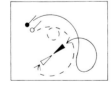

313 a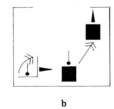

b

c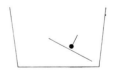

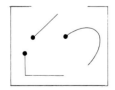

313 d

e

f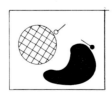

F

Body Signs

Die Körperzeichen

Les signes du corps

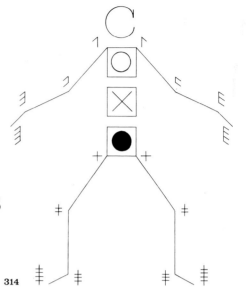

314

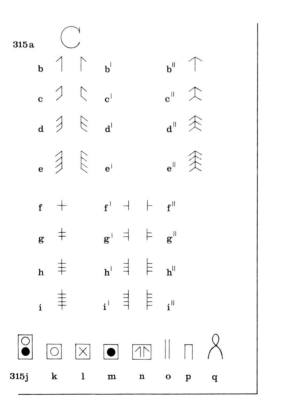

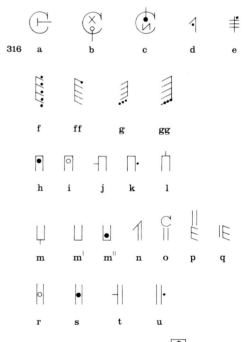

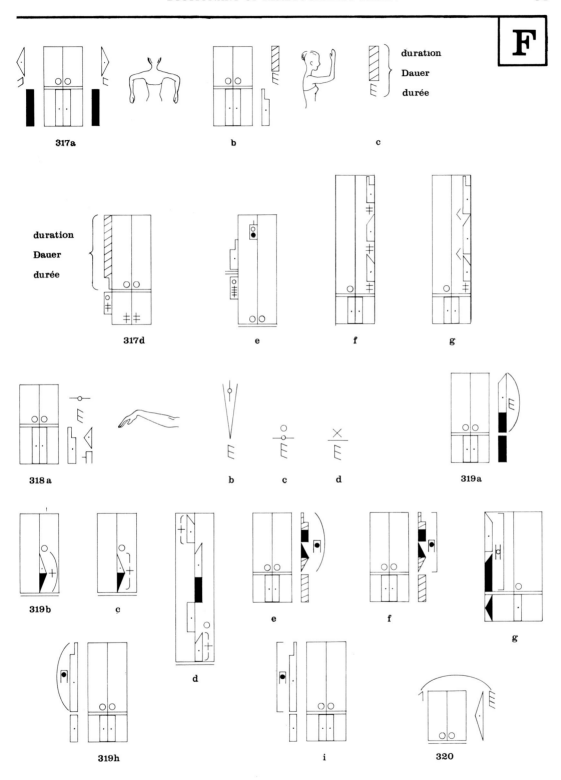

duration
Dauer
durée

317a   b   c

duration
Dauer
durée

317d   e   f   g

318 a   b   c   d   319a

319b   c   d   e   f   g

319h   i   320

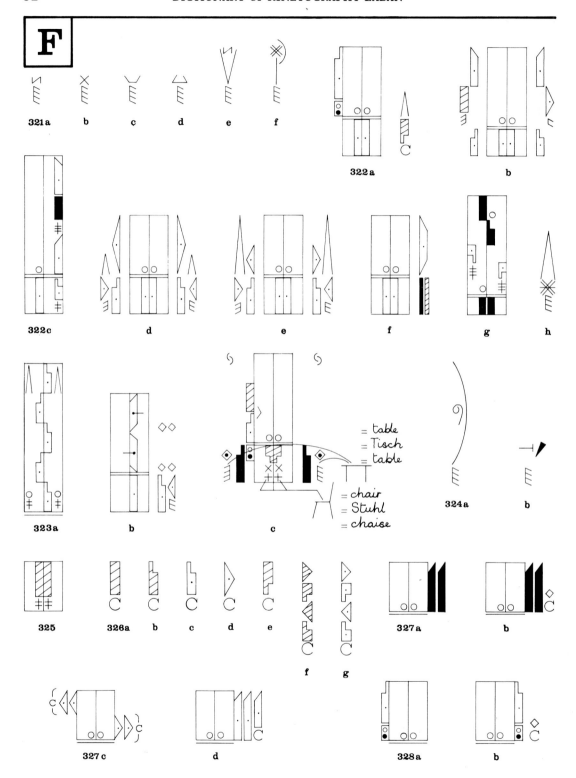

321a   b   c   d   e   f

322a   b

322c   d   e   f   g   h

323a   b   c

= table
= Tisch
= table

= chair
= Stuhl
= chaise

324a   b

325   326a   b   c   d   e   f   g   327a   b

327c   d   328a   b

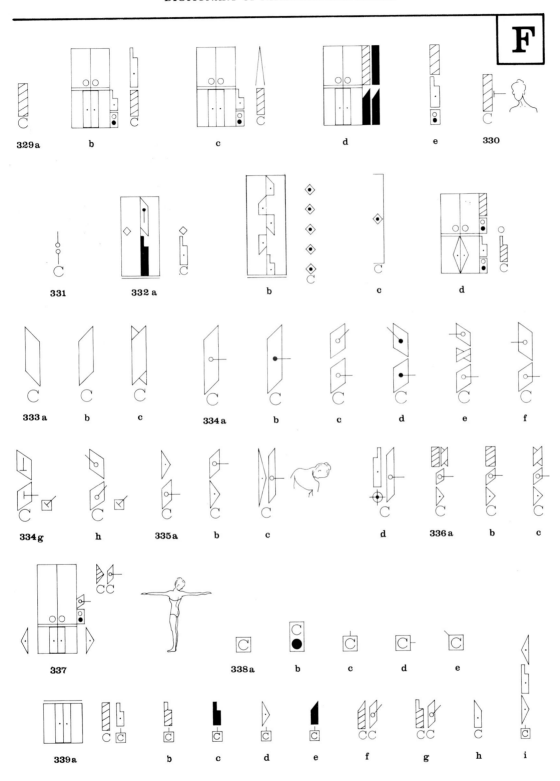

F

329a   b   c   d   e   330

331   332 a   b   c   d

333 a   b   c   334 a   b   c   d   e   f

334 g   h   335 a   b   c   d   336 a   b   c

337   338 a   b   c   d   e

339 a   b   c   d   e   f   g   h   i

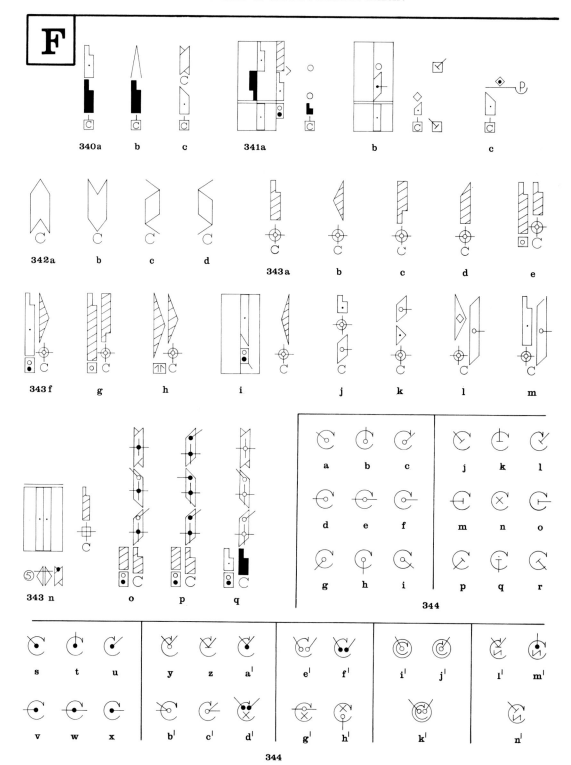

F

340a   b   c   341a   b   c

342a   b   c   d   343a   b   c   d   e

343f   g   h   i   j   k   l   m

343n   o   p   q

a   b   c   j   k   l

d   e   f   m   n   o

g   h   i   p   q   r

344

s   t   u   y   z   a¹   e¹   f¹   i¹   j¹   l¹   m¹

v   w   x   b¹   c¹   d¹   g¹   h¹   k¹   n¹

344

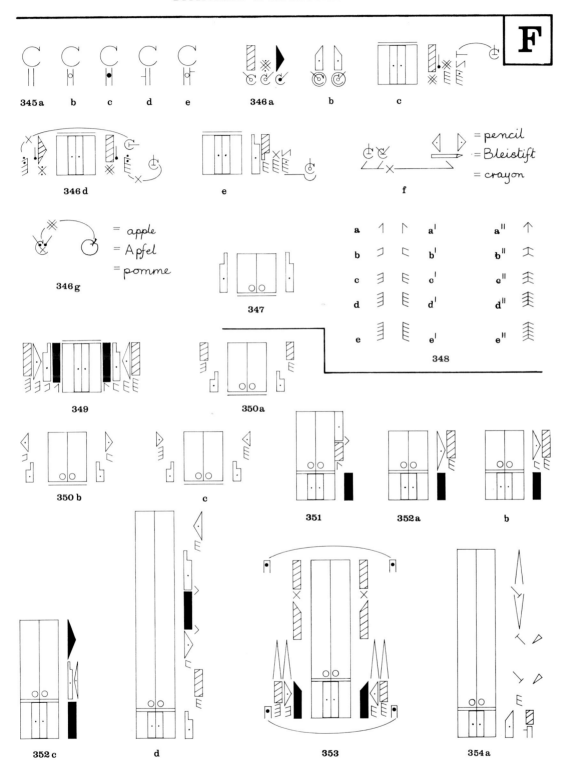

345 a   b   c   d   e   346 a   b   c

346 d   e   f

= pencil
= Bleistift
= crayon

346 g

= apple
= Apfel
= pomme

347

a	⌐	Γ	a'		a''	↑
b			b'		b''	
c			c'		c''	
d			d'		d''	
e			e'		e''	

348

349   350 a

350 b   c   351   352 a   b

352 c   d   353   354 a

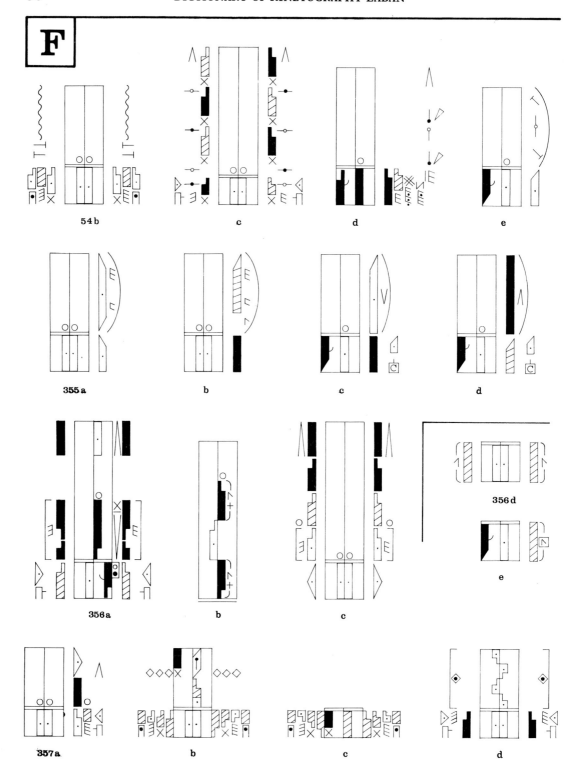

54 b   c   d   e

355 a   b   c   d

356 a   b   c   356 d

e

357 a   b   c   d

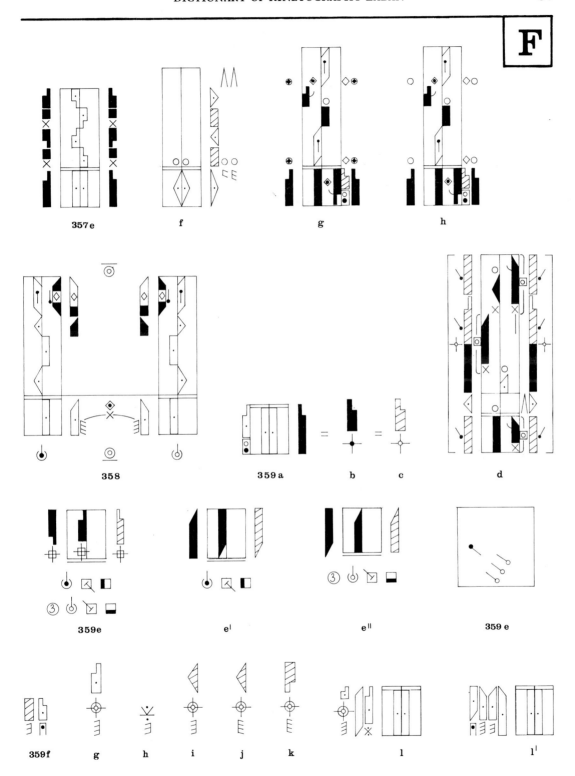

357e   **f**   **g**   **h**

358   **359a**   **b**   **c**   **d**

359e   **e^I**   **e^II**   **359e**

359f   **g**   **h**   **i**   **j**   **k**   **l**   **l^I**

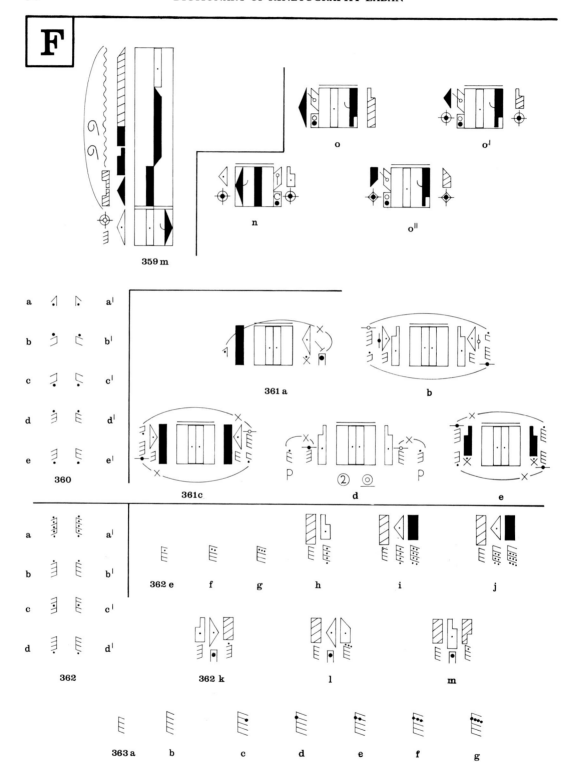

F

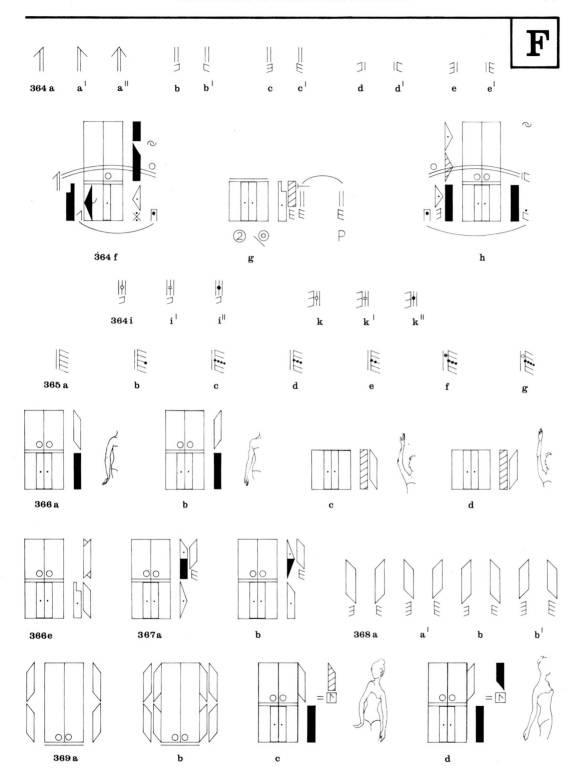

364 a a' a'' b b' c c' d d' e e'

364 f g h

364 i i' i'' k k' k''

365 a b c d e f g

366 a b c d

366 e 367 a b 368 a a' b b'

369 a b c d

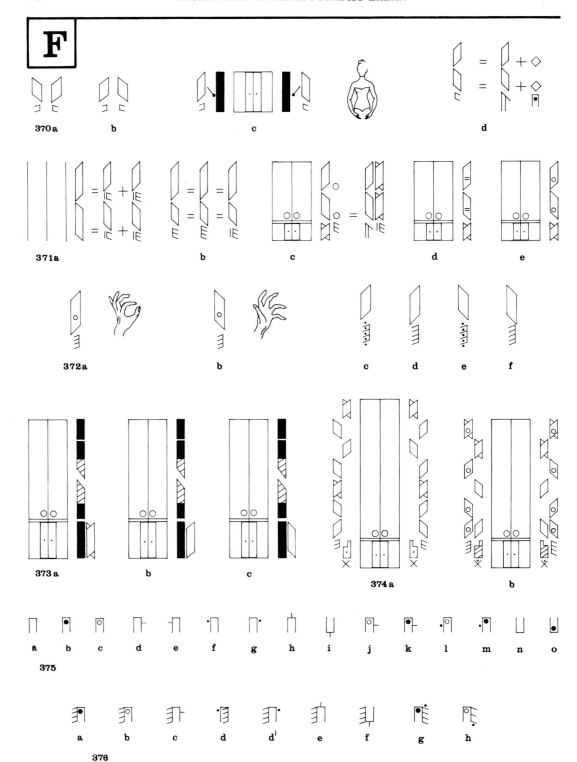

370a   b   c   d

371a   b   c   d   e

372a   b   c   d   e   f

373a   b   c   374a   b

375   a   b   c   d   e   f   g   h   i   j   k   l   m   n   o

376   a   b   c   d   d¹   e   f   g   h

F

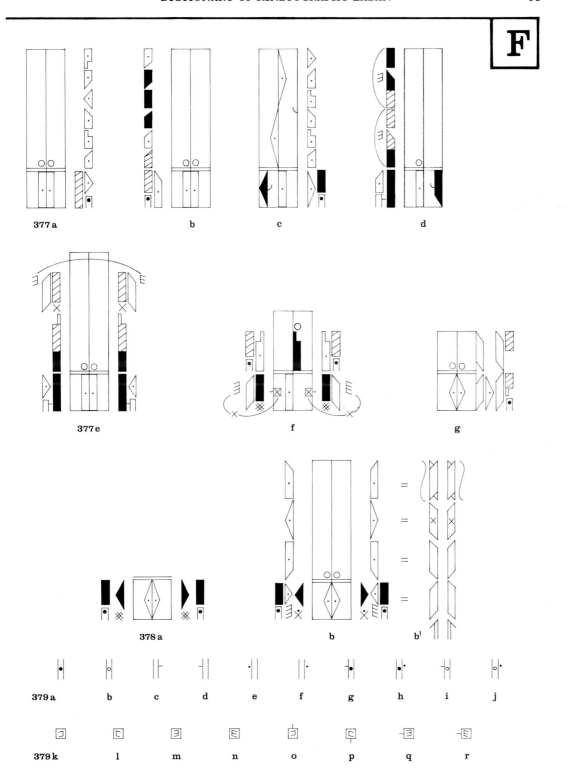

377a   b   c   d

377e   f   g

378a   b   b¹

379a   b   c   d   e   f   g   h   i   j

379k   l   m   n   o   p   q   r

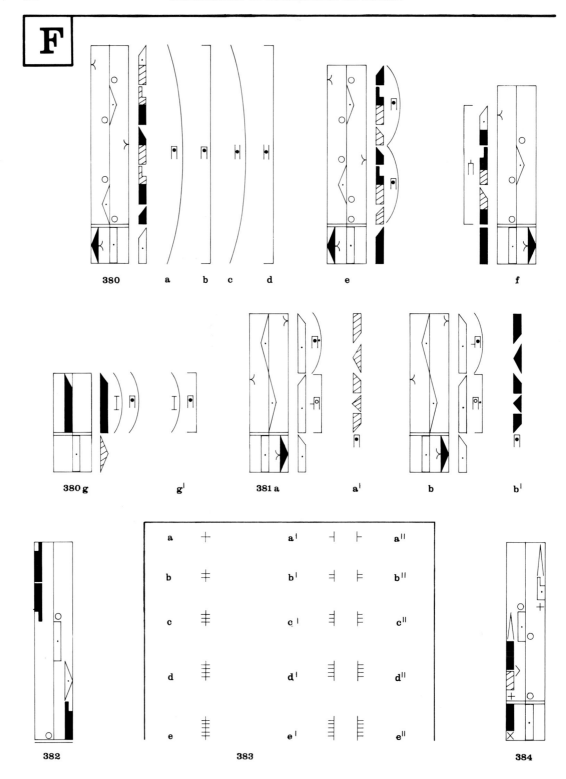

380   a   b   c   d   e   f

380 g   g'   381 a   a'   b   b'

382   383   384

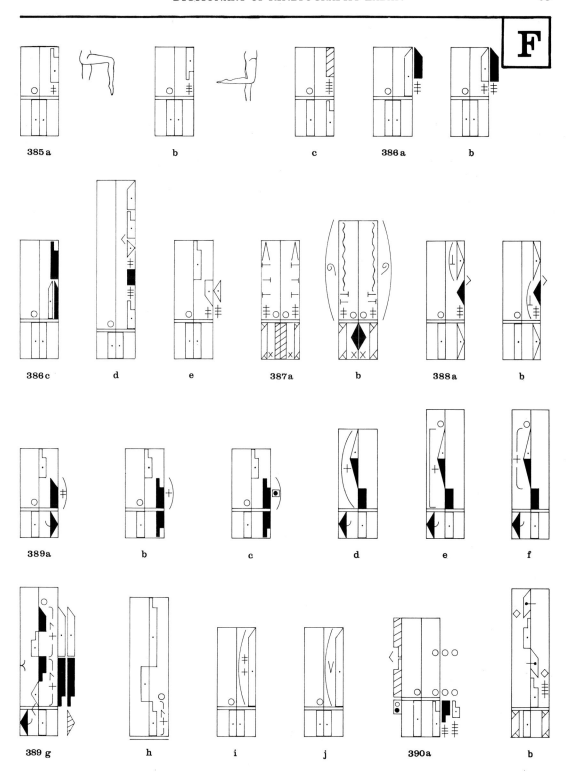

385 a   b   c   386 a   b

386 c   d   e   387 a   b   388 a   b

389a   b   c   d   e   f

389 g   h   i   j   390a   b

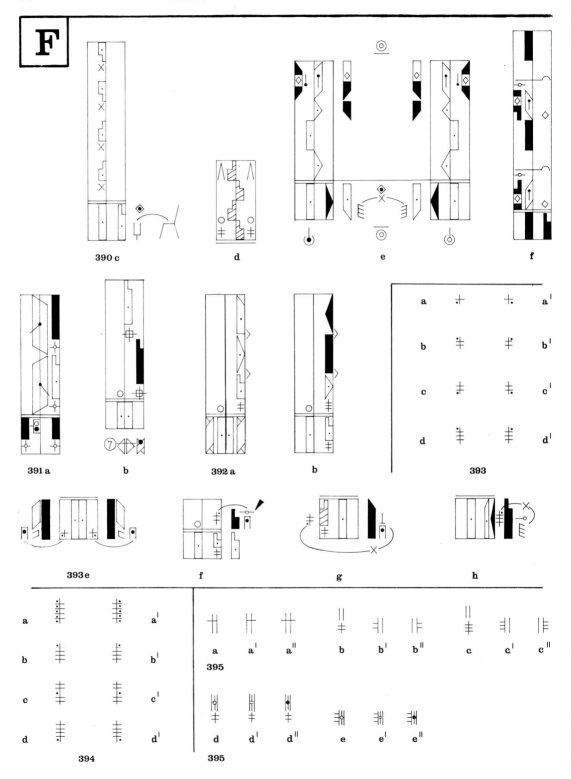

390 c   **d**   **e**   **f**

391 a   **b**   **392 a**   **b**   **393**

393 e   **f**   **g**   **h**

394   **395**

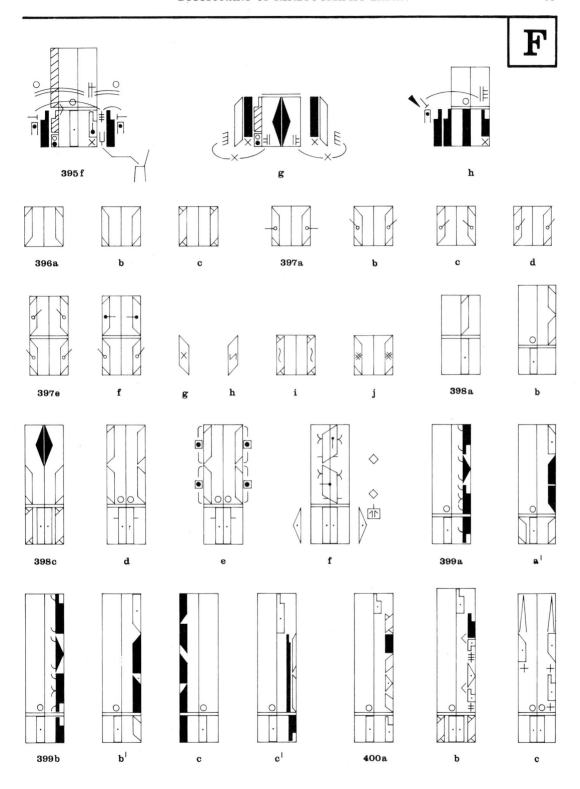

395f

g

h

396a   b   c   397a   b   c   d

397e   f   g   h   i   j   398a   b

398c   d   e   f   399a   a'

399b   b'   c   c'   400a   b   c

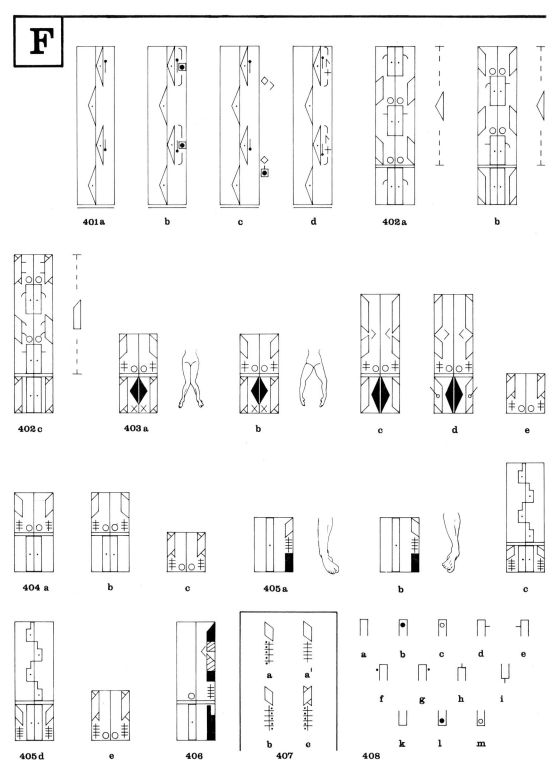

401a   b   c   d   402a   b

402c   403a   b   c   d   e

404a   b   c   405a   b   c

405d   e   406   407   408

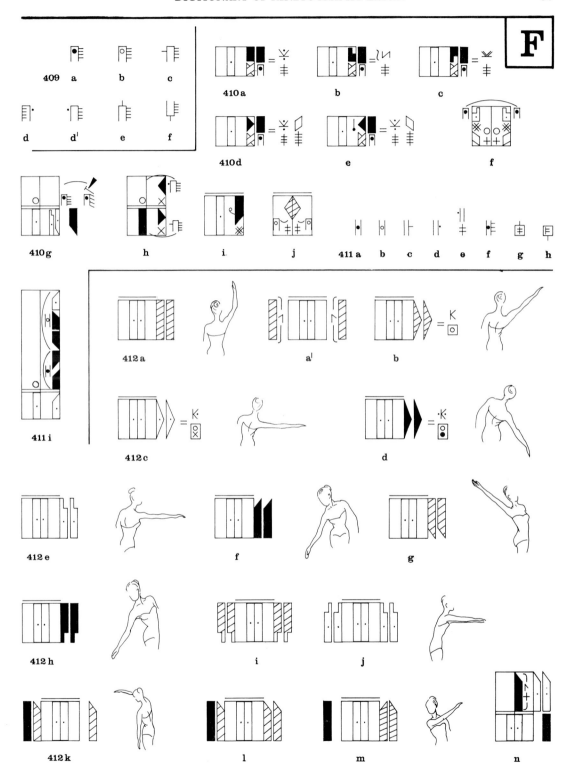

F

409 a b c d d¹ e f

410a b c

410d e f

410g h i j

411a b c d e f g h

411i

412a a¹ b

412c d

412e f g

412h i j

412k l m n

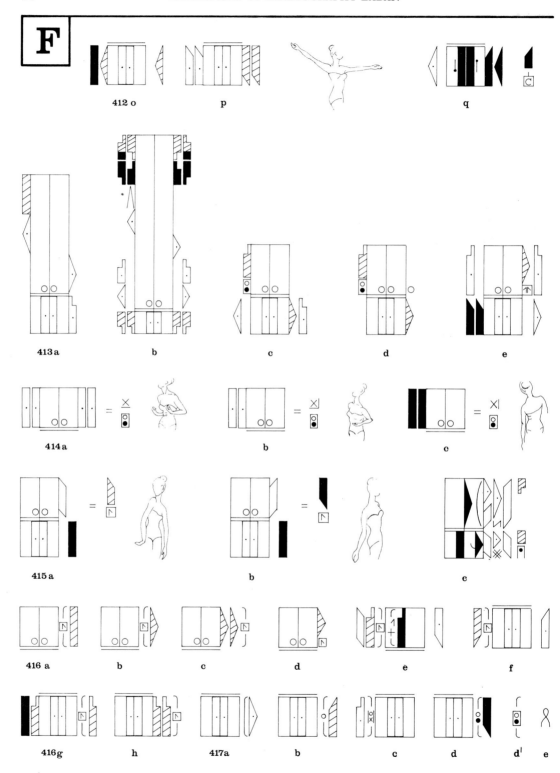

412 o   p   q

413 a   b   c   d   e

414 a   b   c

415 a   b   c

416 a   b   c   d   e   f

416 g   h   417 a   b   c   d   d¹   e

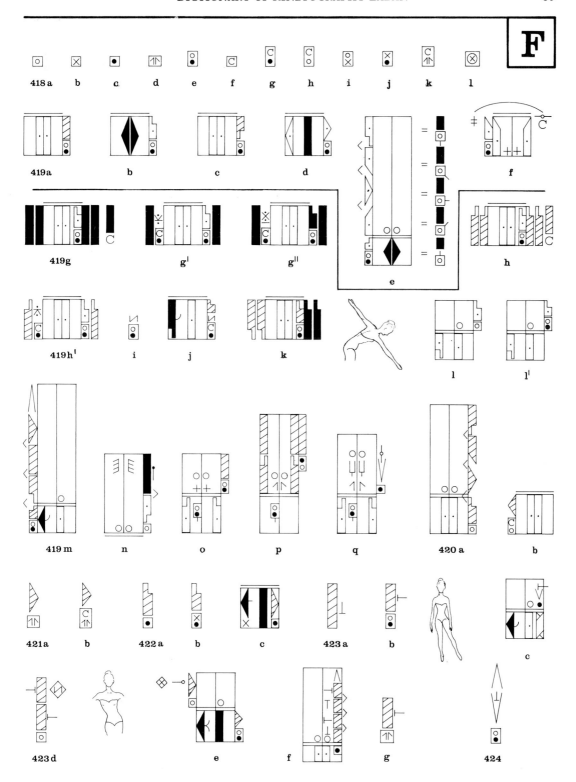

F

418 a   b   c   d   e   f   g   h   i   j   k   l

419a   b   c   d   e   f

419g   g^I   g^II   h

419h^I   i   j   k   l   l^I

419 m   n   o   p   q   420 a   b

421a   b   422 a   b   c   423 a   b   c

423 d   e   f   g   424

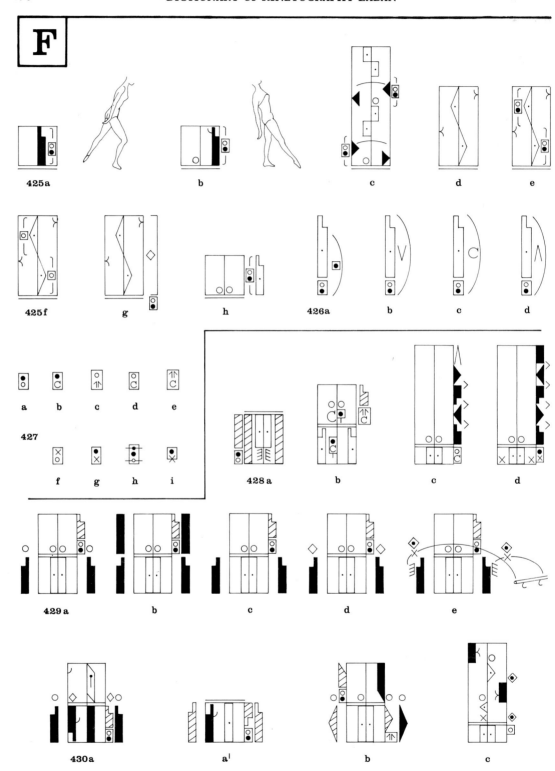

425a
b
c
d
e

425f
g
h
426a
b
c
d

427
a
b
c
d
e

f
g
h
i

428a
b
c
d

429a
b
c
d
e

430a
aᴵ
b
c

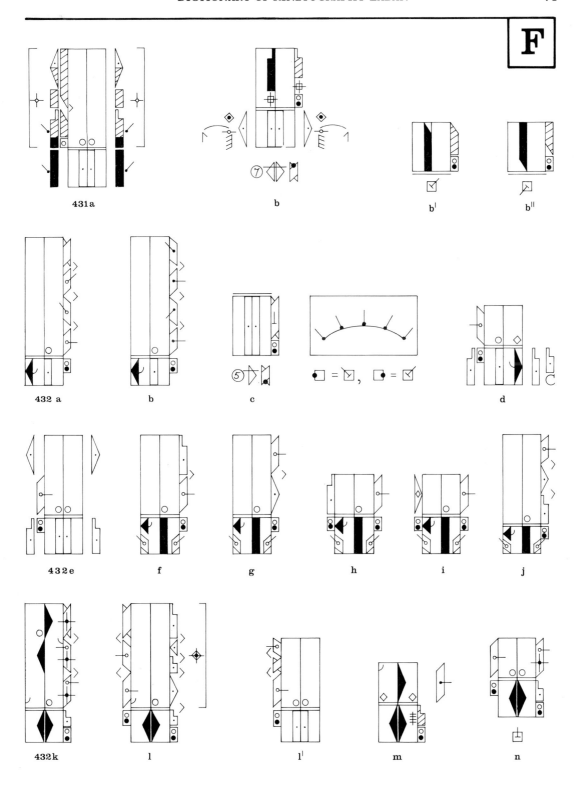

431a   b   b^I b^{II}

432 a b c   d

432e f g h i j

432k l l^I m n

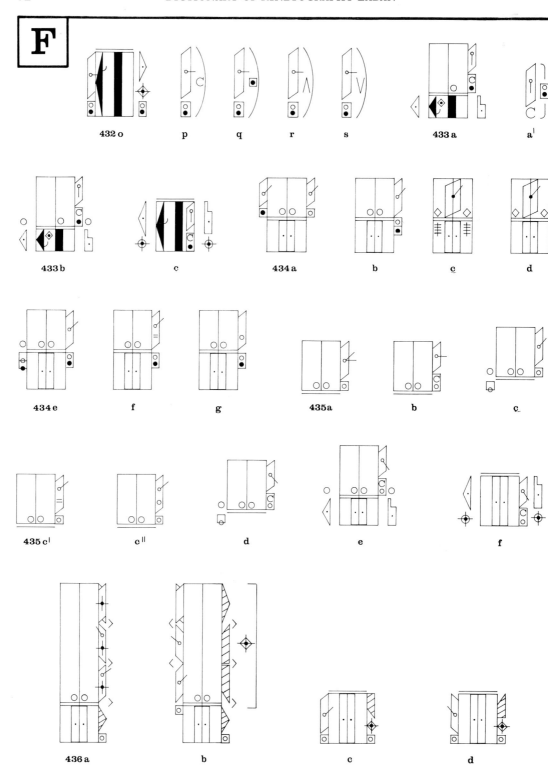

432 o   p   q   r   s   433 a   a¹

433 b   c   434 a   b   c   d

434 e   f   g   435 a   b   c

435 c¹   c¹¹   d   e   f

436 a   b   c   d

F

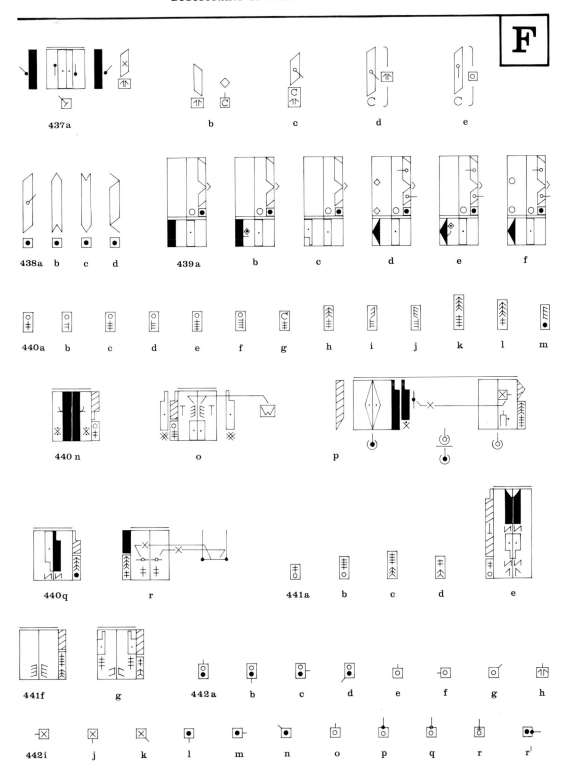

437a   b   c   d   e

438a b c d   439a   b   c   d   e   f

440a b c d e f g h i j k l m

440 n   o   p

440q   r   441a b c d   e

441f   g   442a b c d e f g h

442i   j   k   l   m   n   o   p   q   r   r'

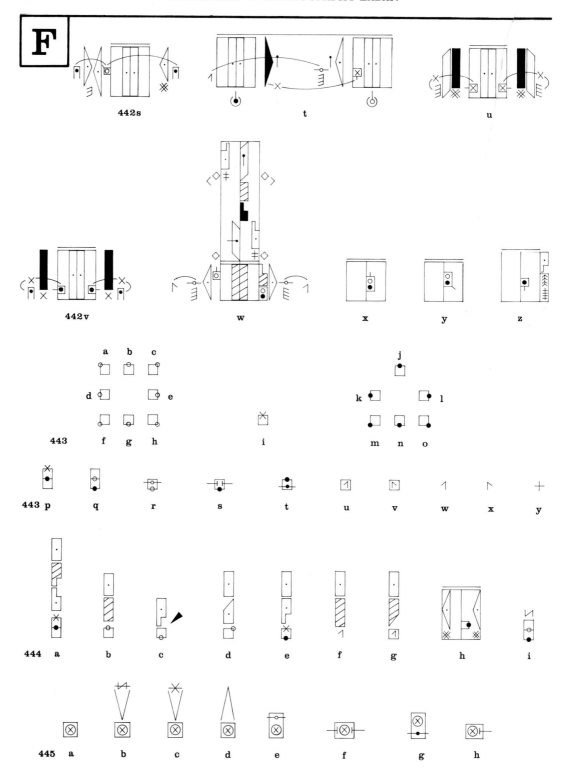

442s

t

u

442v

w

x

y

z

a   b   c

j

d   e

k   l

443   f   g   h   i   m   n   o

443 p   q   r   s   t   u   v   w   x   y

444 a   b   c   d   e   f   g   h   i

445 a   b   c   d   e   f   g   h

Supporting on Parts of the Body
Übertragungen auf die Körperteile
Transferts sur les parties du corps

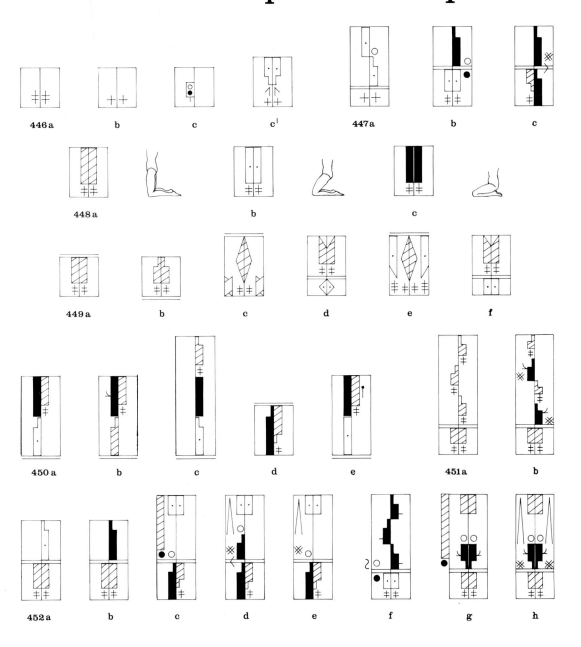

446a   b   c   c¹   447a   b   c

448a   b   c

449a   b   c   d   e   f

450a   b   c   d   e   451a   b

452a   b   c   d   e   f   g   h

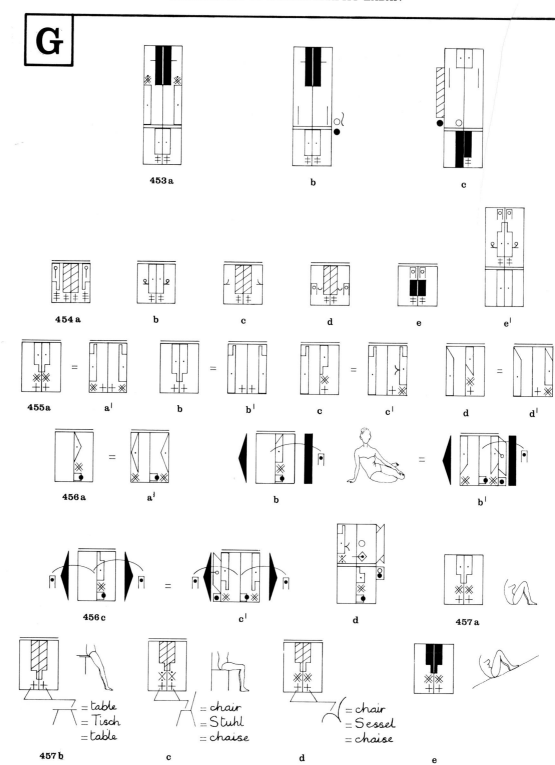

G

453 a   b   c

454 a   b   c   d   e   e¹

455 a   a¹   b   b¹   c   c¹   d   d¹

456 a   a¹   b   b¹

456 c   c¹   d   457 a

457 b   c   d   e

= table
= Tisch
= table

= chair
= Stuhl
= chaise

= chair
= Sessel
= chaise

G

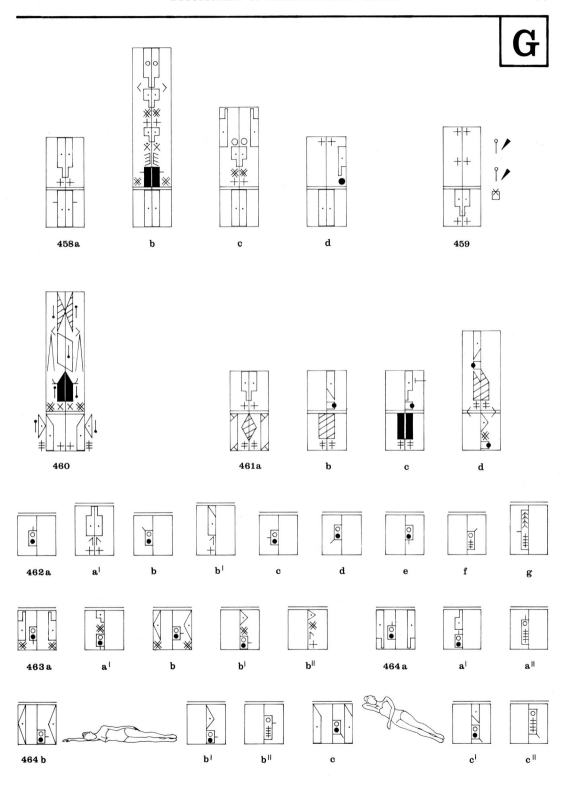

458a   b   c   d   459

460   461a   b   c   d

462a   a^I   b   b^I   c   d   e   f   g

463a   a^I   b   b^I   b^{II}   464a   a^I   a^{II}

464b   b^I   b^{II}   c   c^I   c^{II}

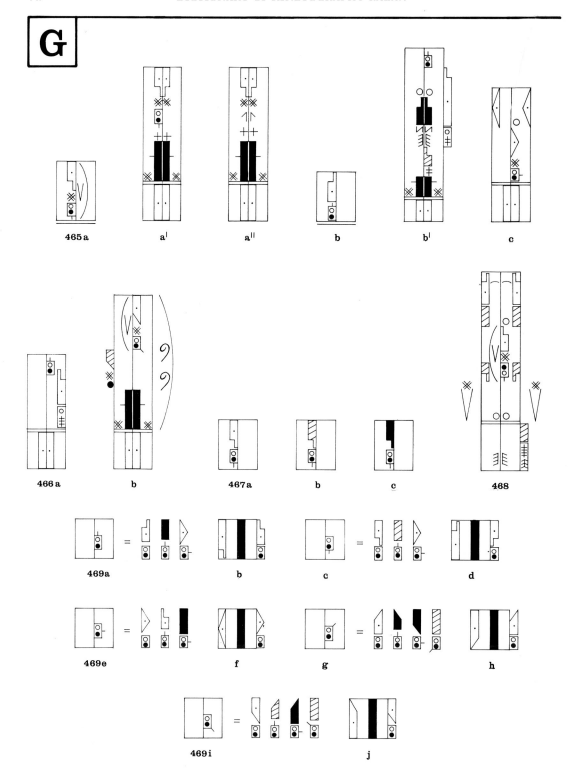

465a   a^I   a^{II}   b   b^I   c

466a   b   467a   b   c   468

469a   b   c   d

469e   f   g   h

469i   j

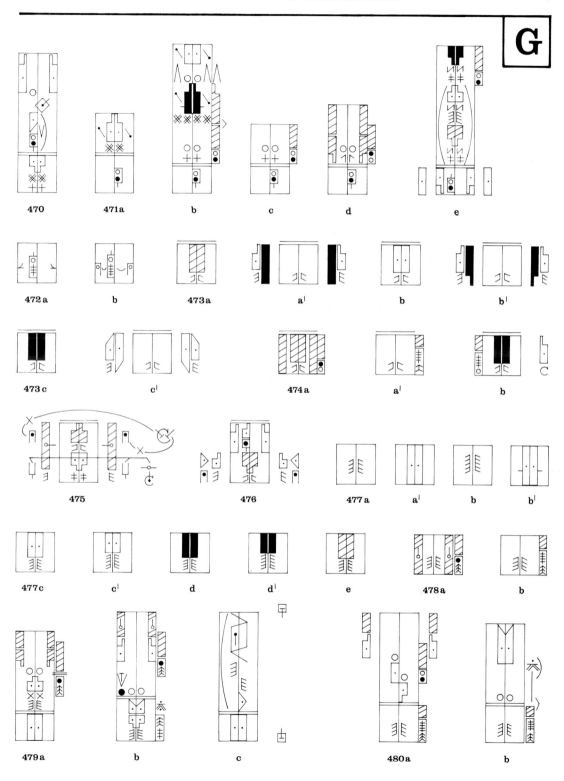

470   471a   b   c   d   e

472a   b   473a   a¹   b   b¹

473c   c¹   474a   a¹   b

475   476   477a   a¹   b   b¹

477c   c¹   d   d¹   e   478a   b

479a   b   c   480a   b

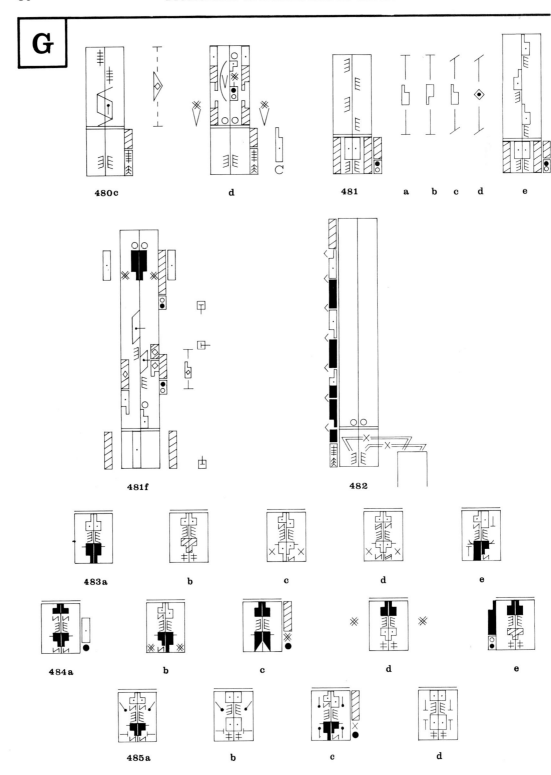

480c

d

481 a b c d e

481f

482

483a b c d e

484a b c d e

485a b c d

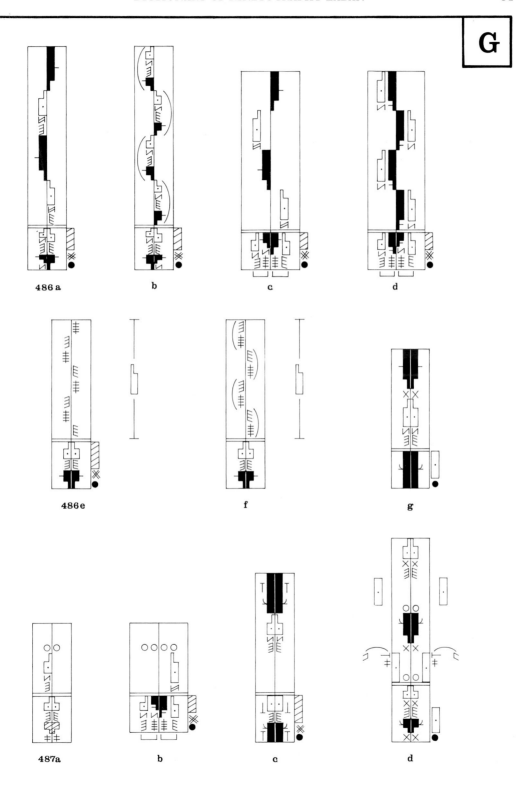

486 a   b   c   d

486 e   f   g

487a   b   c   d

G

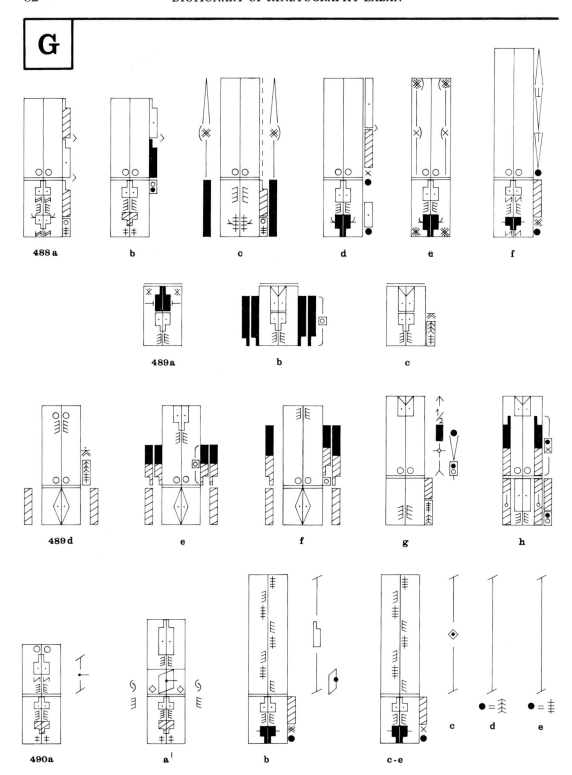

488 a   b   c   d   e   f

489a   b   c

489 d   e   f   g   h

490a   a'   b   c-e

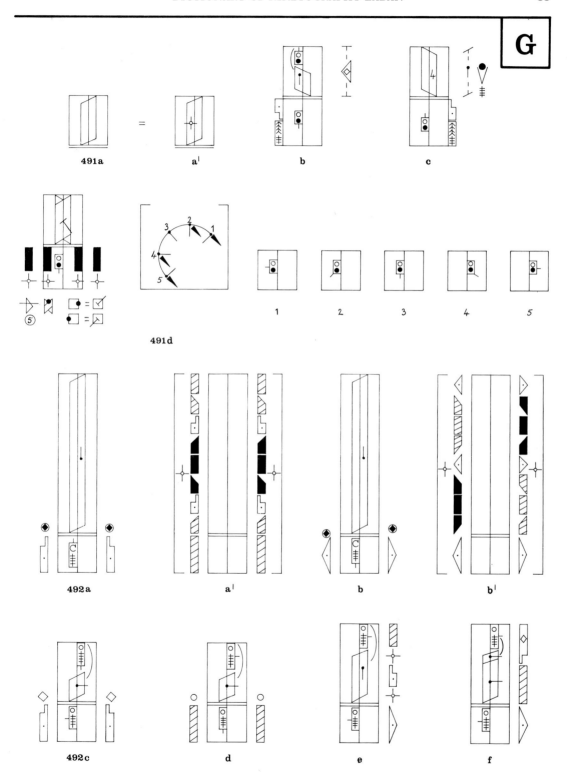

491a   a'   b   c

491d

1   2   3   4   5

492a   a'   b   b'

492c   d   e   f

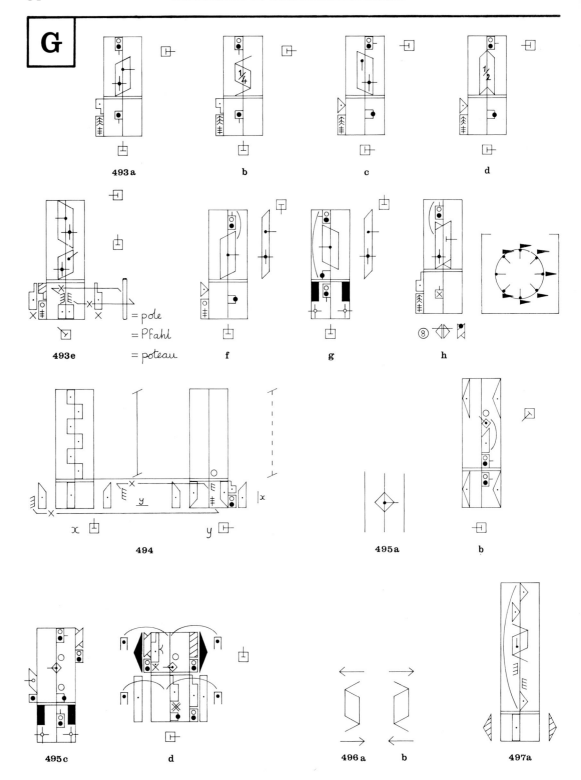

G

493 a   b   c   d

= pole
= Pfahl
= poteau

493 e   f   g   h

494   495 a   b

495 c   d   496 a   b   497a

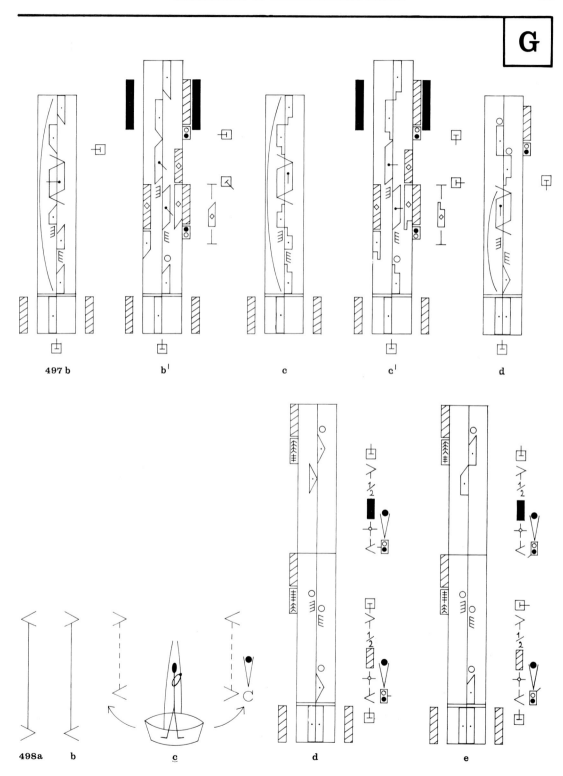

497 b   b¹   c   c¹   d

498a   b   c   d   e

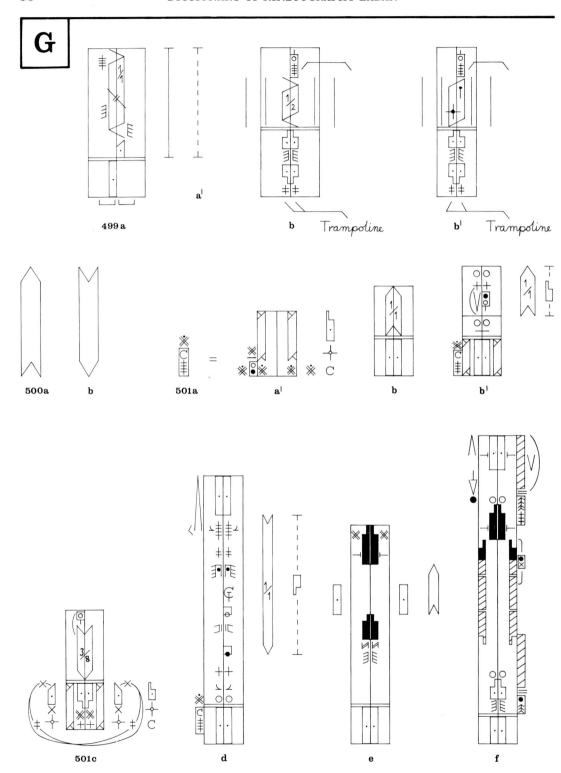

G

499 a   b   *Trampoline*   b¹   *Trampoline*

500a   b   501a   a¹   b   b¹

501c   d   e   f

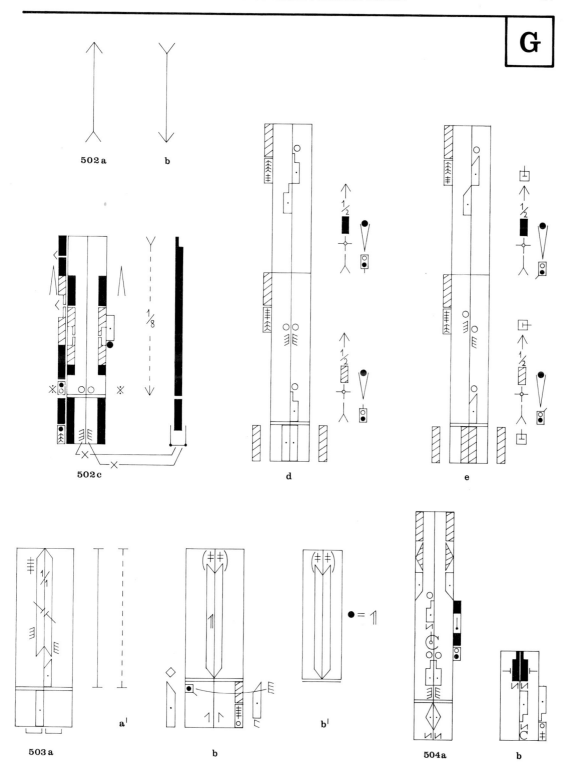

502 a   b

502 c   d   e

503 a   a'   b   b'   504a   b

G

$\boxed{A}$ = aqua $\boxed{AE}$ = aequor $\boxed{T}$ = terra

505 a   b   c

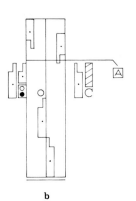

b

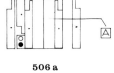

506 a

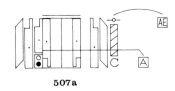

507 a

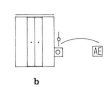

b

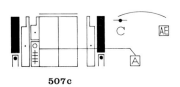

507 c

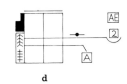

d

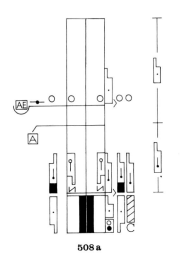

508 a

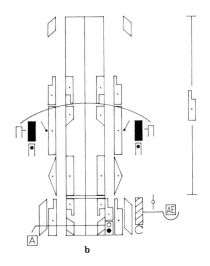

b

The Centre of Gravity
Schwerpunktbewegungen
Mouvements du centre de gravité

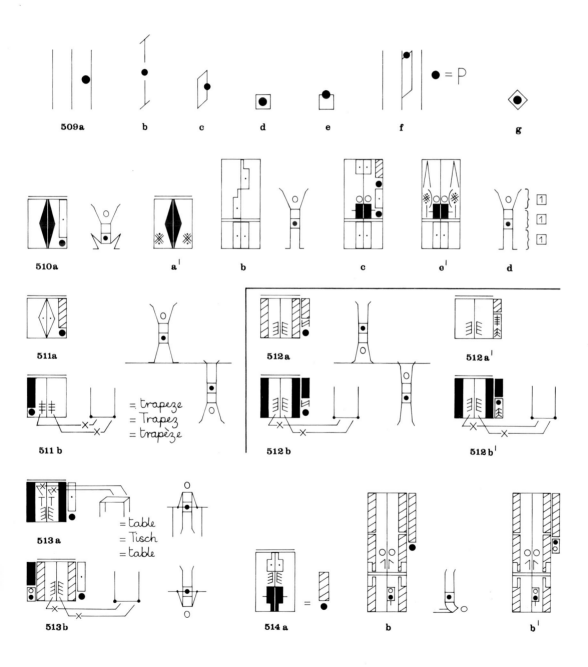

509a   b   c   d   e   f   g

510a   a¹   b   c   c¹   d

511a

= trapeze
= Trapez
= trapèze

511 b

512a   512a¹

512 b   512b¹

513a

= table
= Tisch
= table

513b

514 a   b   b¹

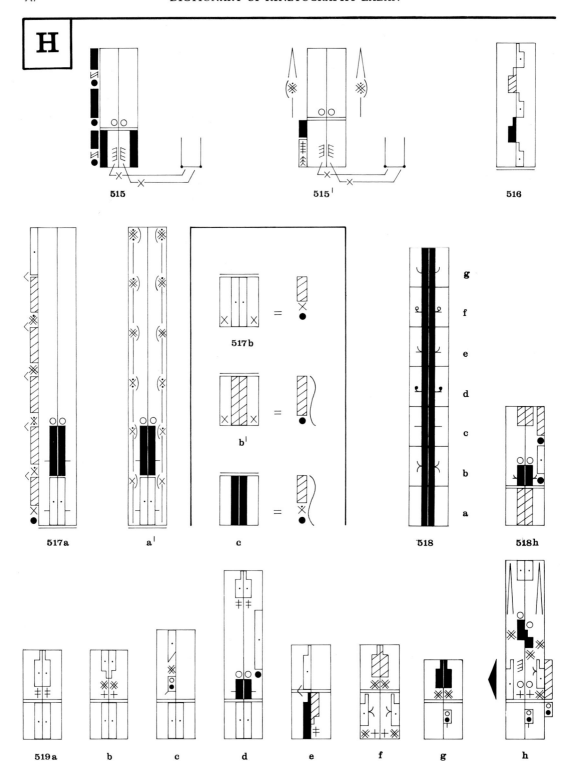

515

515'

516

517a

a'

517b

b'

c

518

518h

519a   b   c   d   e   f   g   h

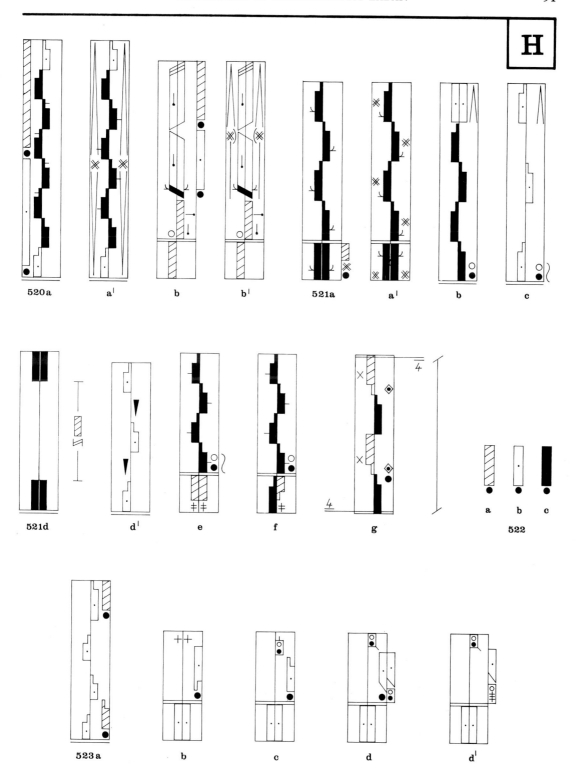

520a   a¹   b   b¹   521a   a¹   b   c

521d   d¹   e   f   g   a   b   c

522

523a   b   c   d   d¹

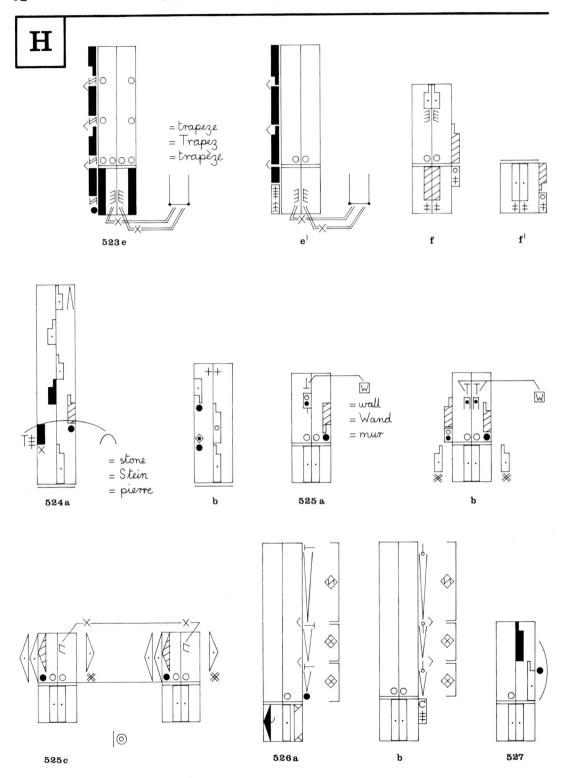

= trapeze
= Trapez
= trapèze

523 e   **e¹**   **f**   **f¹**

= stone
= Stein
= pierre

524 a   **b**

= wall
= Wand
= mur

525 a   **b**

525 c   **526 a**   **b**   **527**

Relation Signs
Die Beziehungszeichen
Les signes de relation

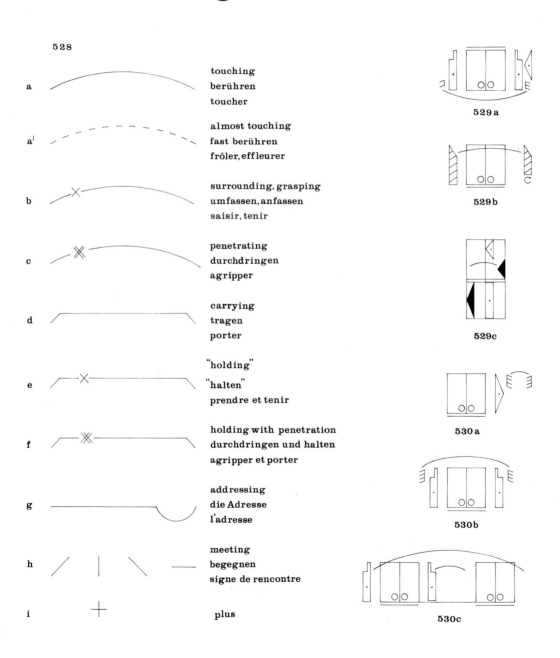

528

a — touching / berühren / toucher

529a

a' — almost touching / fast berühren / frôler, effleurer

529b

b — surrounding, grasping / umfassen, anfassen / saisir, tenir

c — penetrating / durchdringen / agripper

529c

d — carrying / tragen / porter

e — "holding" / "halten" / prendre et tenir

530a

f — holding with penetration / durchdringen und halten / agripper et porter

g — addressing / die Adresse / l'adresse

530b

h — meeting / begegnen / signe de rencontre

i — plus

530c

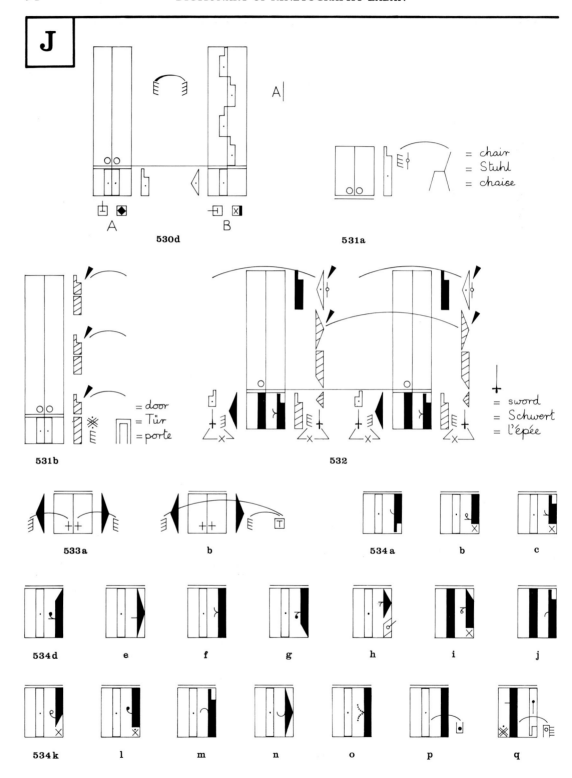

J

530d

531a

= chair
= Stuhl
= chaise

531b

= door
= Tür
= porte

532

= sword
= Schwert
= l'épée

533a   b   534a   b   c

534d   e   f   g   h   i   j

534k   l   m   n   o   p   q

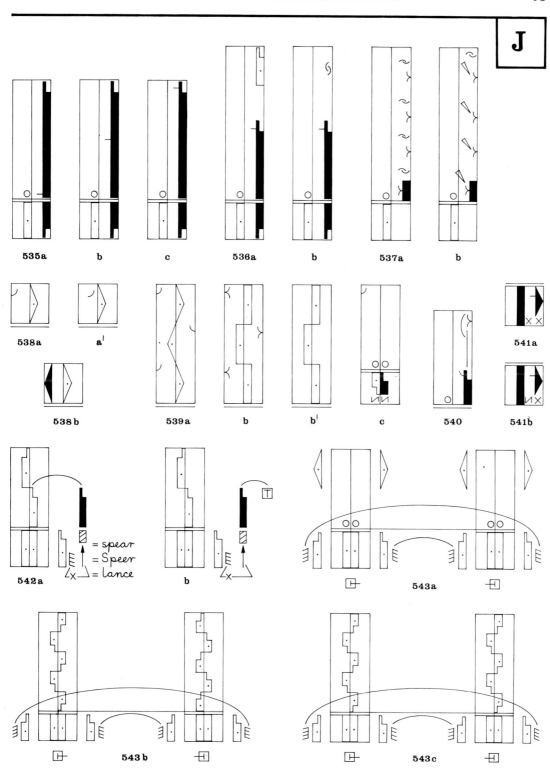

535a   b   c   536a   b   537a   b

538a   a¹

538b   539a   b   b¹   c   540   541b

541a

= spear
= Speer
= lance

542a   b   543a

543b   543c

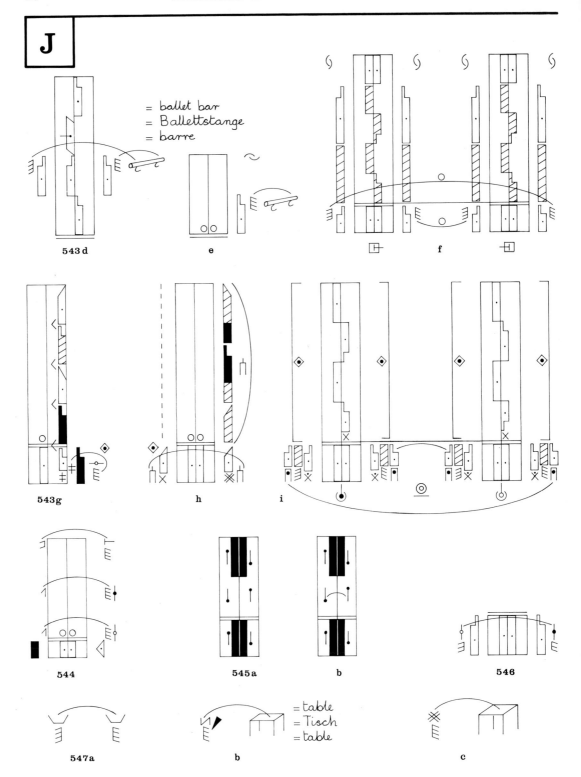

= ballet bar
= Ballettstange
= barre

543 d

e

f

543g

h

i

544

545a

b

546

547a

b

= table
= Tisch
= table

c

J

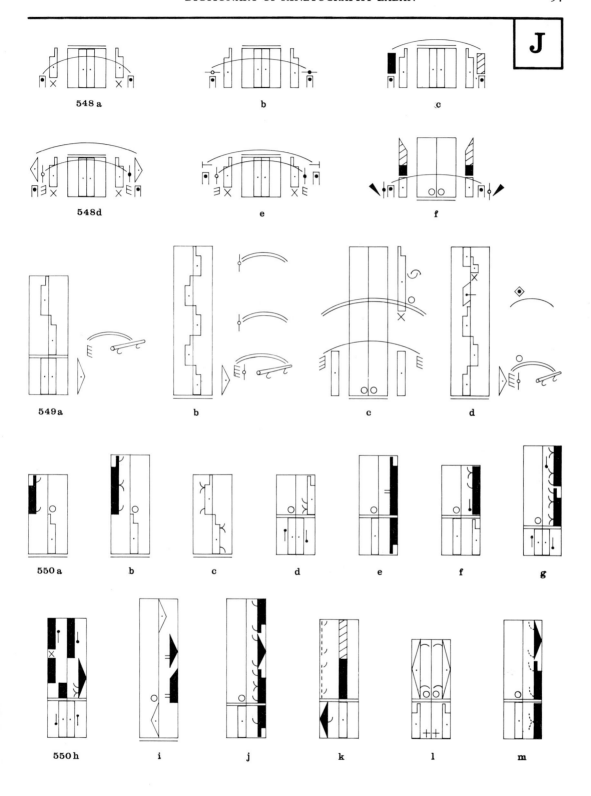

548 a   b   c

548 d   e   f

549 a   b   c   d

550 a   b   c   d   e   f   g

550 h   i   j   k   l   m

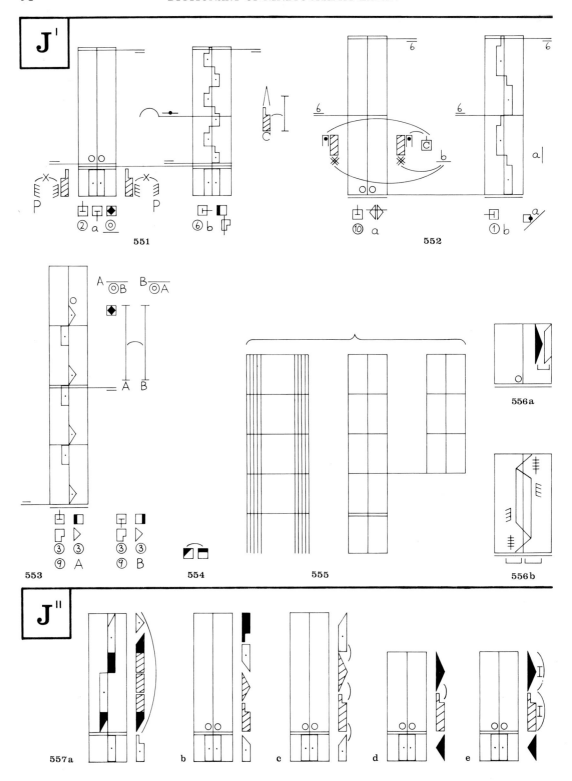

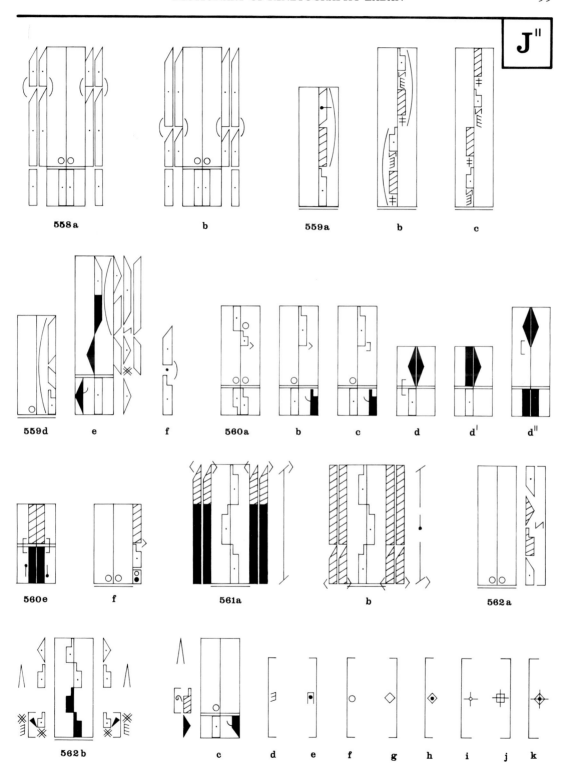

558a   b   559a   b   c

559d   e   f   560a   b   c   d   d^{I} d^{II}

560e   f   561a   b   562a

562b   c   d   e   f   g   h   i   j   k

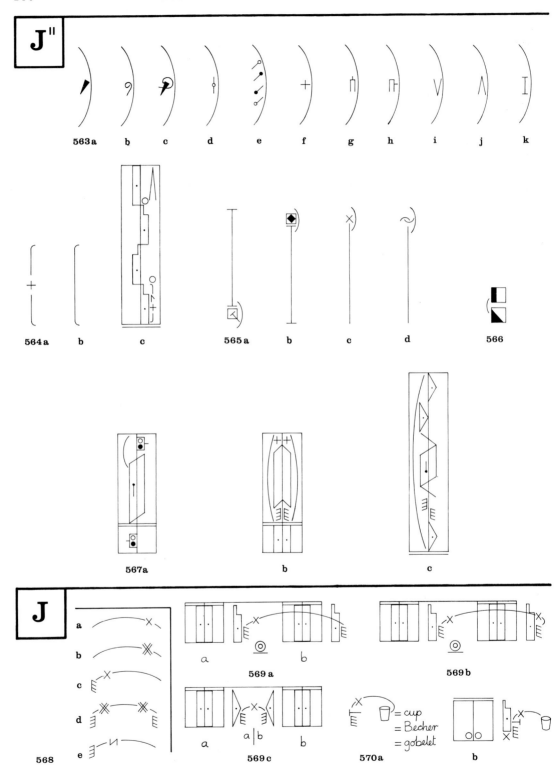

J"

563a b c d e f g h i j k

564a b c 565a b c d 566

567a b c

J

a b c d e

568

569a a b

569b

569c a|b b

570a = cup = Becher = gobelet

b

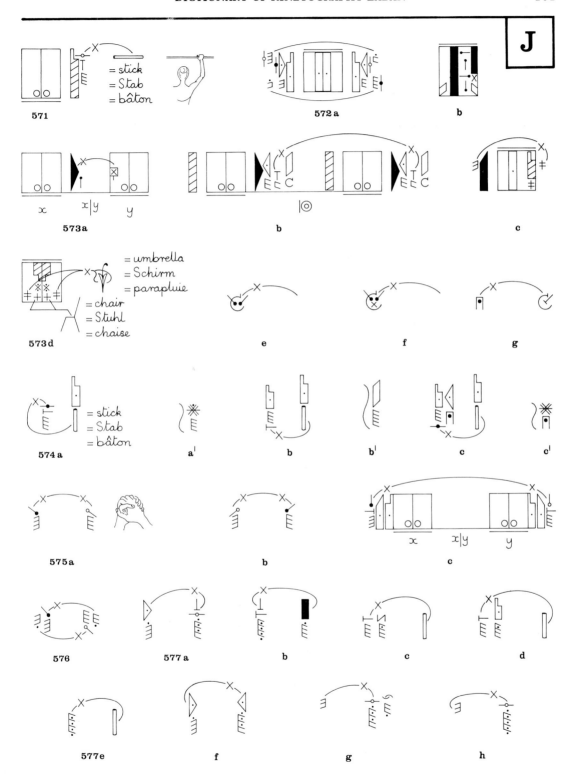

= stick
= Stab
= bâton

571   **572 a**   **b**   **J**

573a   **b**   **c**

= umbrella
= Schirm
= parapluie

= chair
= Stuhl
= chaise

573d   **e**   **f**   **g**

= stick
= Stab
= bâton

574 a   **a¹**   **b**   **b¹**   **c**   **c¹**

575a   **b**   **c**

576   **577 a**   **b**   **c**   **d**

577e   **f**   **g**   **h**

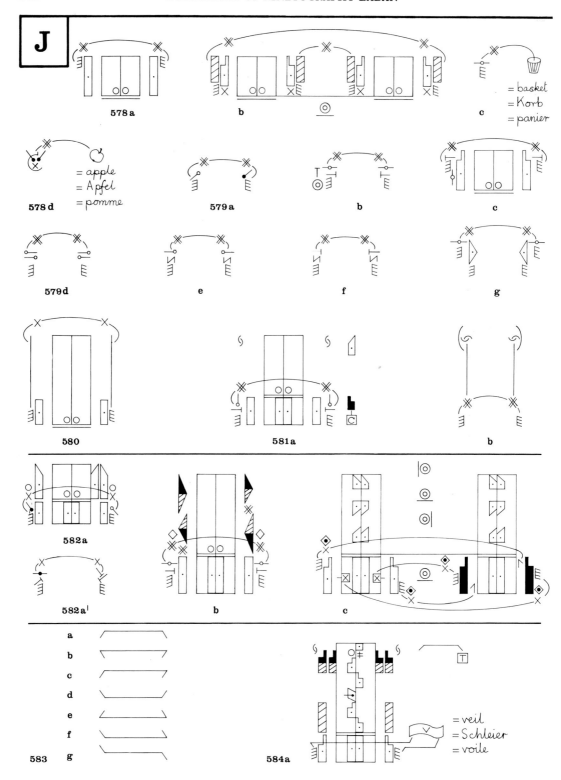

J

578 a

b

c
= basket
= Korb
= panier

578 d
= apple
= Apfel
= pomme

579 a

b

c

579 d

e

f

g

580

581a

b

582a

582a'

b

c

583
a
b
c
d
e
f
g

584a
= veil
= Schleier
= voile

J

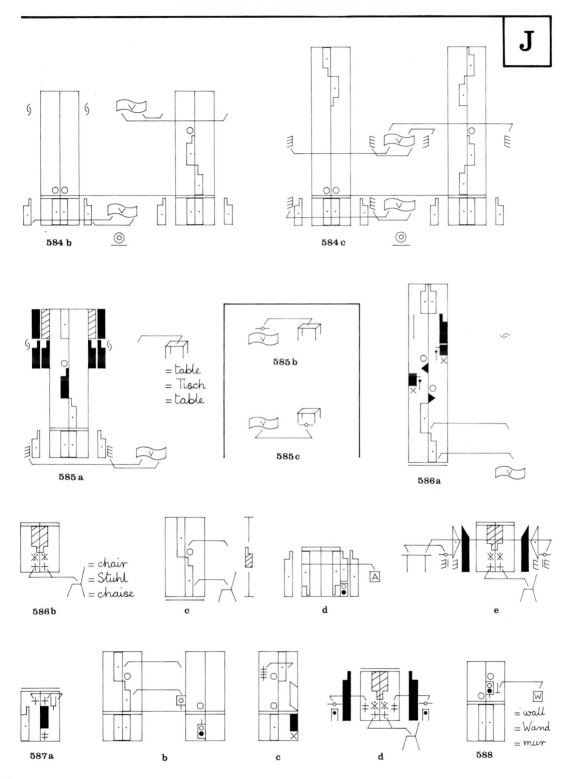

584 b

584 c

585 a

= table
= Tisch
= table

585 b

585 c

586 a

586 b

= chair
= Stuhl
= chaise

c

d

e

587 a

b

c

d

588

= wall
= Wand
= mur

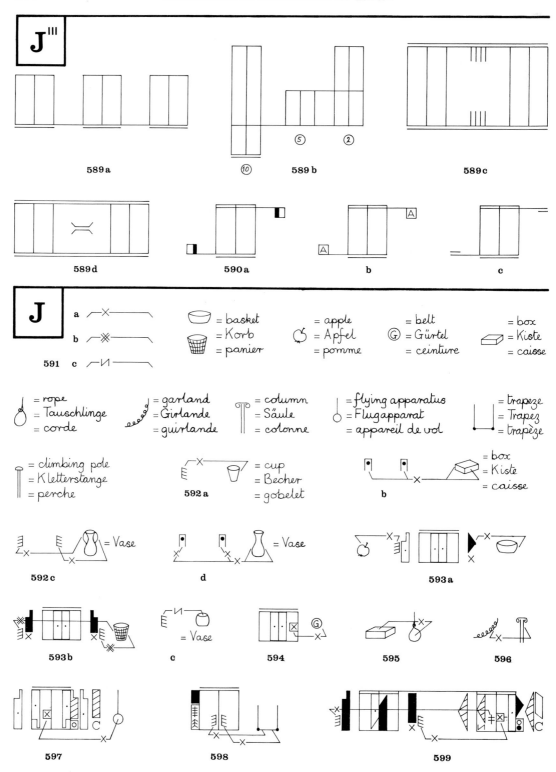

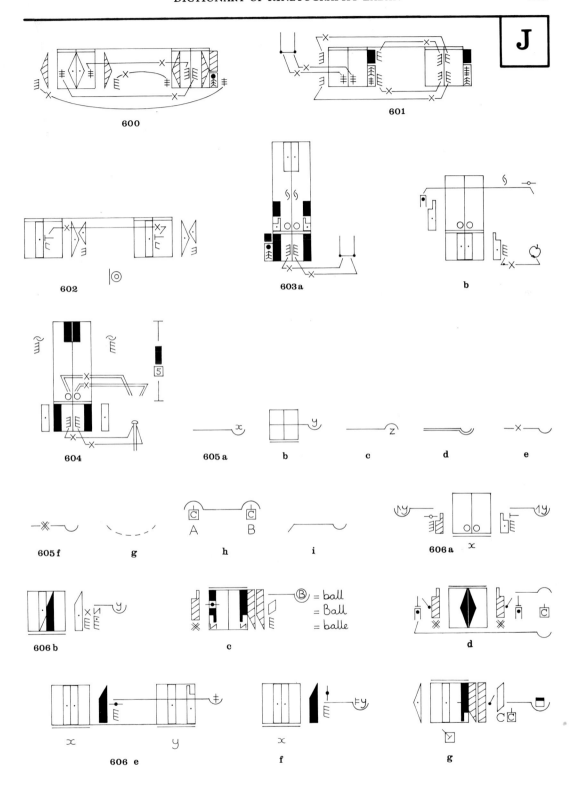

600

601

602

603 a

b

604

605 a

b

c

d

e

605 f

g

h

i

606 a

606 b

c

= ball
= Ball
= balle

d

606 e

f

g

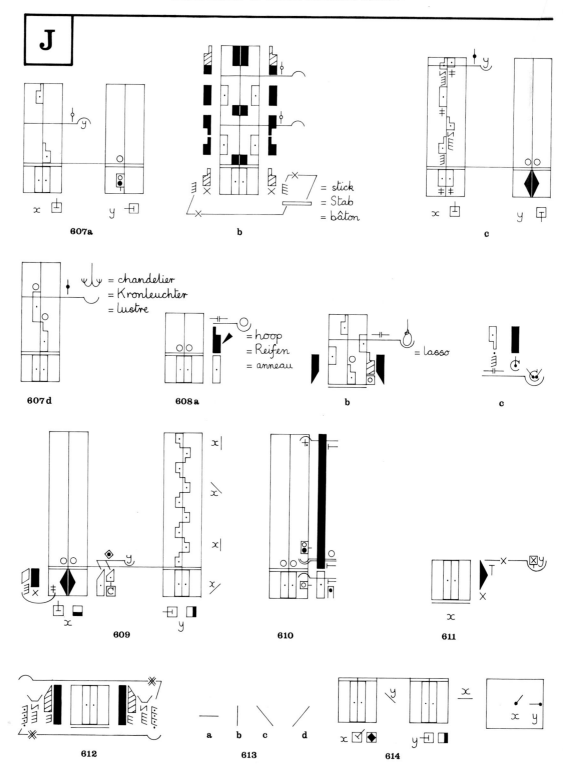

= stick
= Stab
= bâton

607a   b   c

= chandelier
= Kronleuchter
= lustre

= hoop
= Reifen
= anneau

= lasso

607d   608a   b   c

609   610   611

612   613   614

a   b   c   d

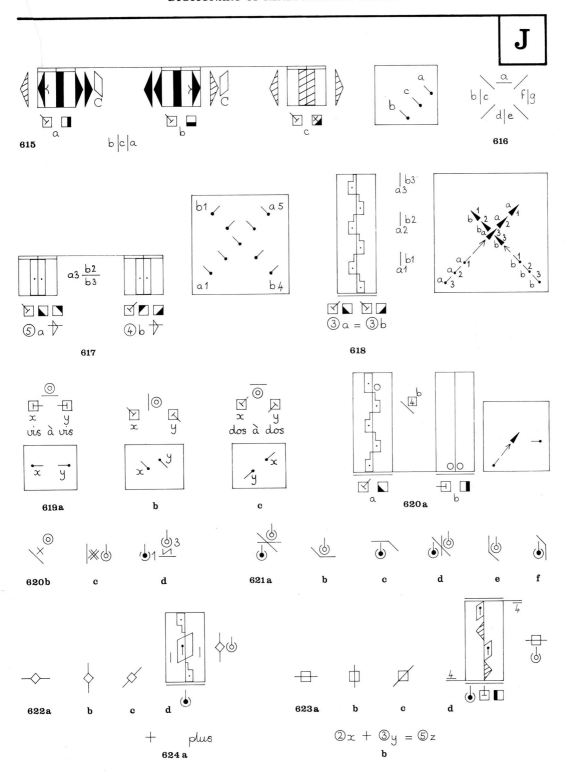

J

615   a   b | c | a   b   c   616

617   a3 $\frac{b2}{b3}$ 618

619a   b   c   620a

620b   c   d   621a   b   c   d   e   f

622a   b   c   d   623a   b   c   d

+   plus

624a $②x + ③y = ⑤z$

b

K Movements of Objects
Die Bewegungen von Gegenständen
Mouvements d'objects

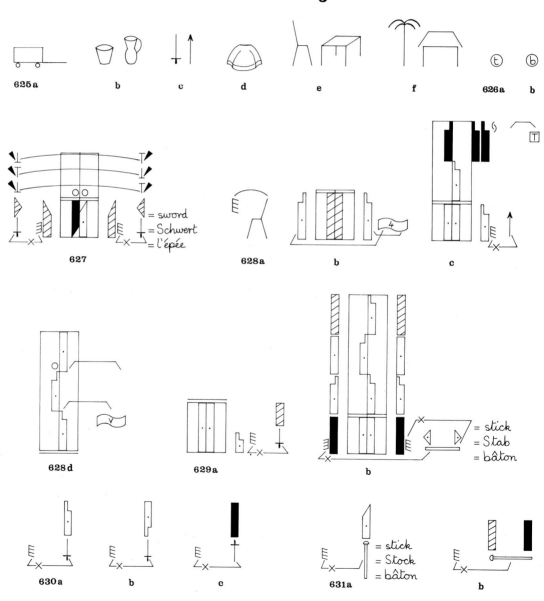

K

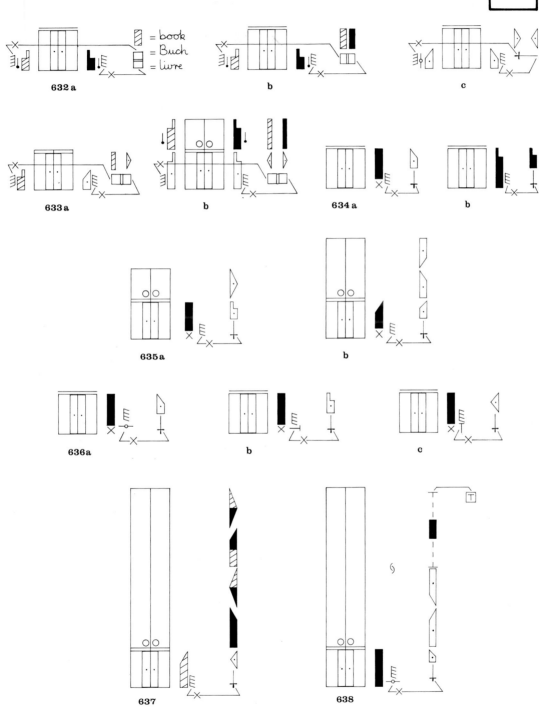

= book
= Buch
= livre

632 a   b   c

633 a   b   634 a   b

635 a   b

636a   b   c

637   638

Quantity Signs
Die Quantitätszeichen
Les signes de quantité

 Space Measurement Signs
Die Raummasszeichen
Les signes d'amplitude (mesure de l'espace)

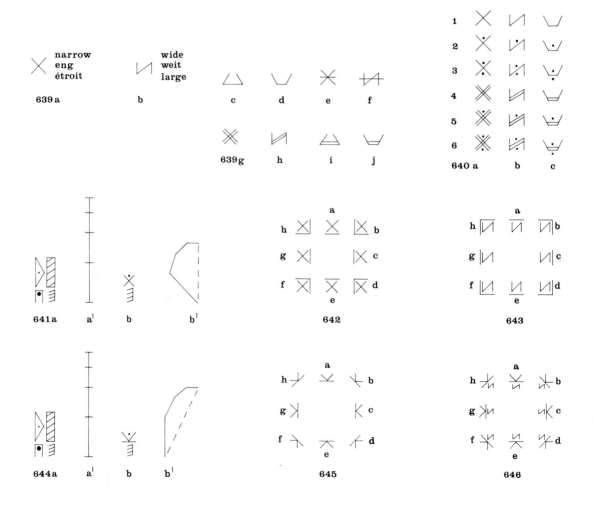

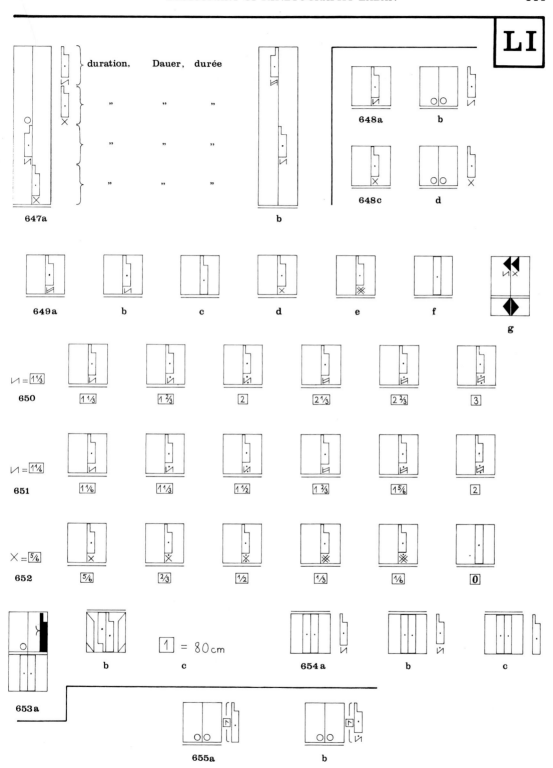

LI

duration, Dauer, durée

647a   b   648a   b   648c   d

649a   b   c   d   e   f   g

$\vee = \boxed{1\frac{1}{3}}$
650        $\boxed{1\frac{1}{3}}$ $\boxed{1\frac{2}{3}}$ $\boxed{2}$ $\boxed{2\frac{1}{3}}$ $\boxed{2\frac{2}{3}}$ $\boxed{3}$

$\vee = \boxed{1\frac{1}{6}}$
651        $\boxed{1\frac{1}{6}}$ $\boxed{1\frac{1}{3}}$ $\boxed{1\frac{1}{2}}$ $\boxed{1\frac{2}{3}}$ $\boxed{1\frac{5}{6}}$ $\boxed{2}$

$\times = \boxed{\frac{5}{6}}$
652        $\boxed{\frac{5}{6}}$ $\boxed{\frac{2}{3}}$ $\boxed{\frac{1}{2}}$ $\boxed{\frac{1}{3}}$ $\boxed{\frac{1}{6}}$ $\boxed{0}$

b   c $\boxed{1} = 80\,cm$ 654a   b   c

653a

655a   b

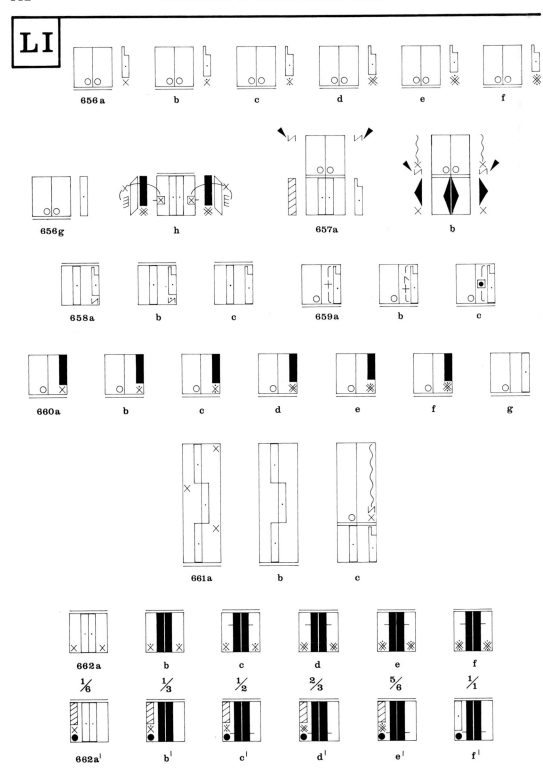

LI

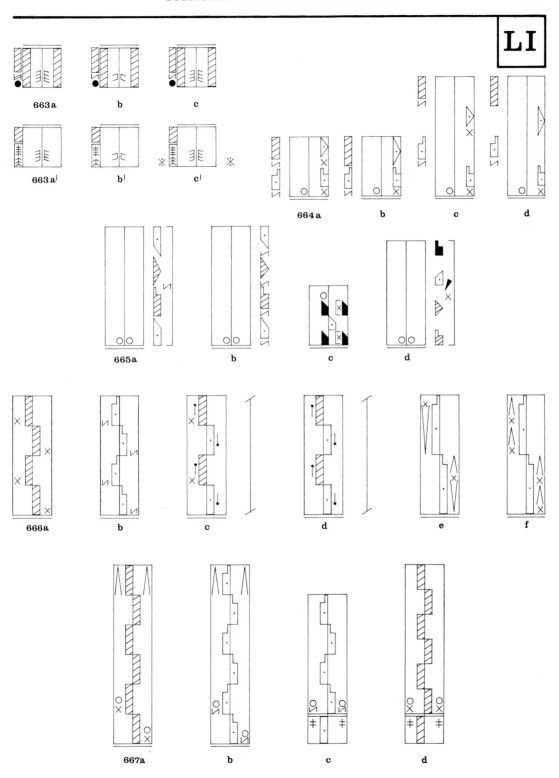

663a   b   c

663 a¹   b¹   c¹

664a   b   c   d

665a   b   c   d

666a   b   c   d   e   f

667a   b   c   d

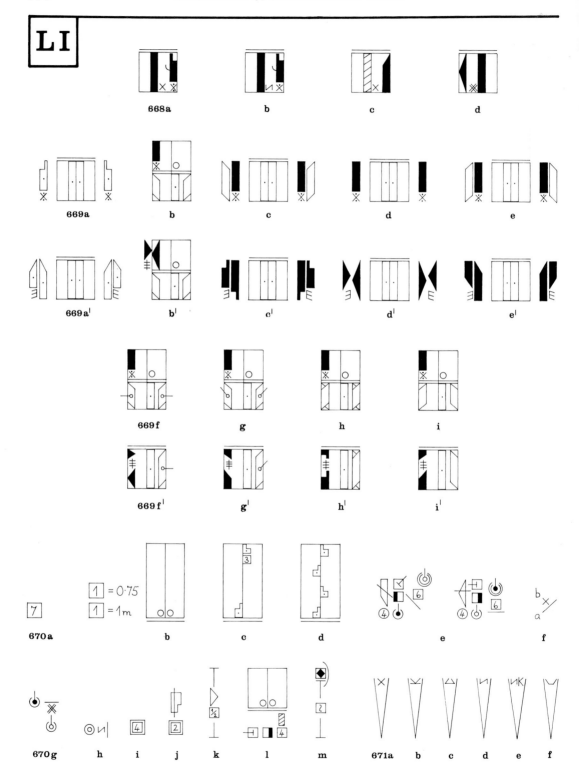

LI

668a   b   c   d

669a   b   c   d   e

669a¹   b¹   c¹   d¹   e¹

669f   g   h   i

669f¹   g¹   h¹   i¹

670a   b   c   d   e   f

$\boxed{1} = 0.75$

$\boxed{1} = 1m$

670g   h   i   j   k   l   m   671a   b   c   d   e   f

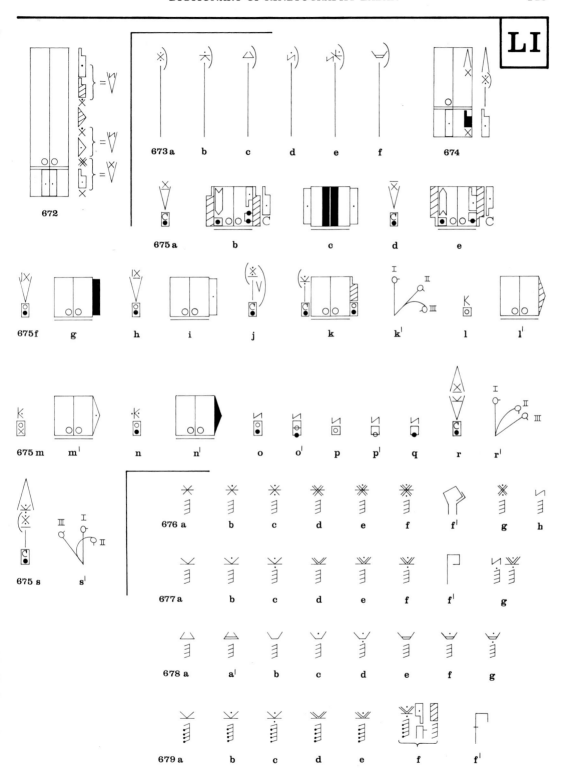

LI

672

673 a   b   c   d   e   f   674

675 a   b   c   d   e

675 f   g   h   i   j   k   k'   l   l'

675 m   m'   n   n'   o   o'   p   p'   q   r   r'

675 s   s'

676 a   b   c   d   e   f   f'   g   h

677 a   b   c   d   e   f   f'   g

678 a   a'   b   c   d   e   f   g

679 a   b   c   d   e   f   f'

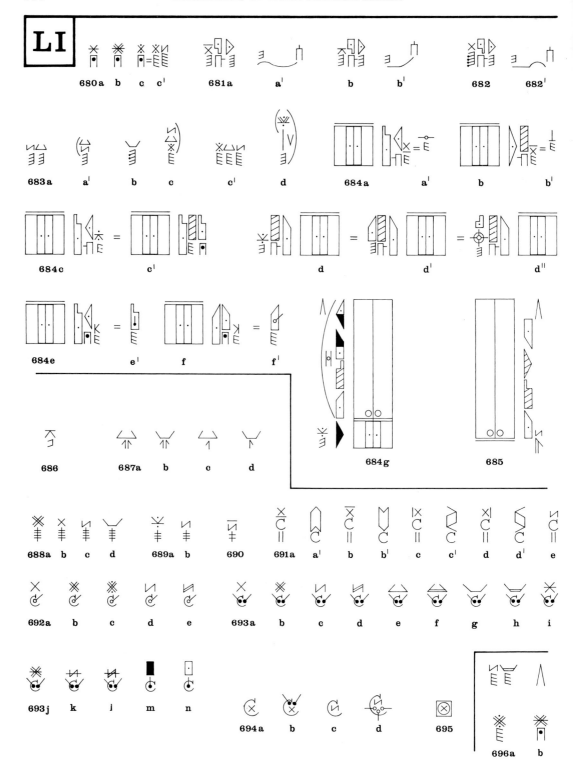

LI

680a b c c¹   681a   a¹   b   b¹   682   682¹

683a a¹ b c   c¹   d   684a   a¹   b   b¹

684c   c¹   d   d¹   d¹¹

684e   e¹   f   f¹   684g   685

686   687a b c d

688a b c d   689a b   690   691a a¹ b b¹ c c¹ d d¹ e

692a b c d e   693a b c d e f g h i

693j k l m n   694a b c d   695   696a b

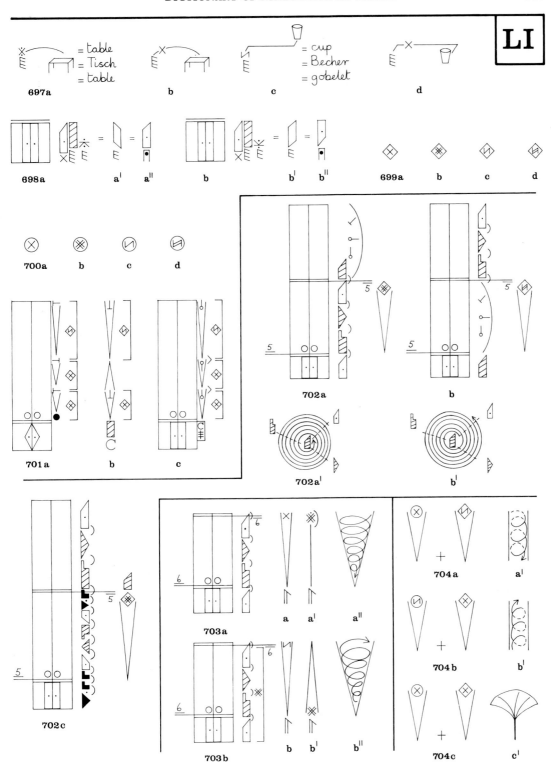

= table
= Tisch
= table

697a   b   c   = cup / = Becher / = gobelet   d

698a   a'   a''   b   b'   b''   699a   b   c   d

700a   b   c   d

701a   b   c

702a   b

702a'   b'

702c

703a   a   a'   a''

703b   b   b'   b''

704a   a'

704b   b'

704c   c'

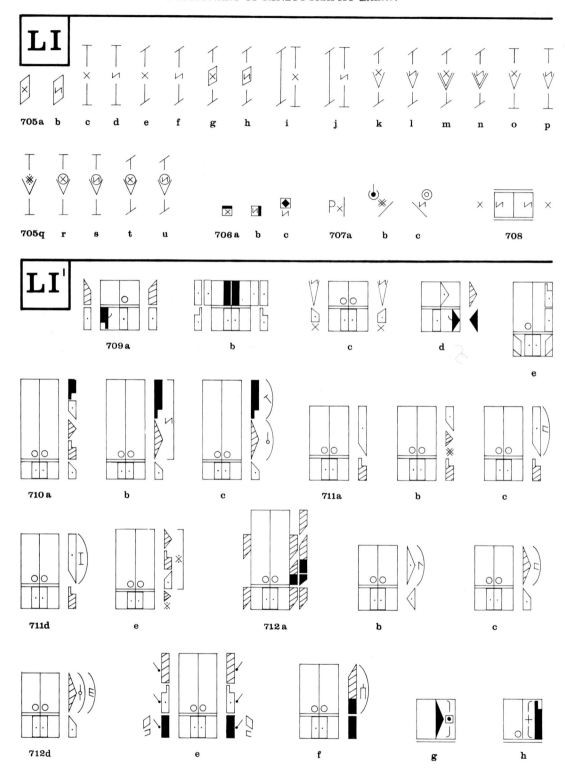

LI

705a   b   c   d   e   f   g   h   i   j   k   l   m   n   o   p

705q   r   s   t   u   706a   b   c   707a   b   c   708

LI¹

709a   b   c   d

e

710a   b   c   711a   b   c

711d   e   712a   b   c

712d   e   f   g   h

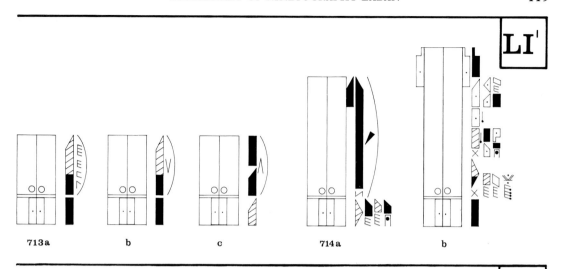

LI'

| 713a | b | c | 714a | b |

Strength Measurement Signs LII

Die Kraftmasszeichen

Les signes dynamiques (mesure de la force)

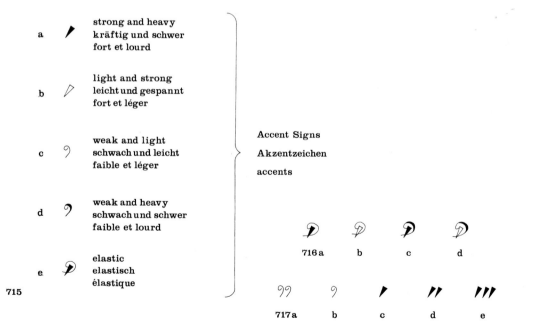

a   strong and heavy
kräftig und schwer
fort et lourd

b   light and strong
leicht und gespannt
fort et léger

c   weak and light
schwach und leicht
faible et léger

d   weak and heavy
schwach und schwer
faible et lourd

e   elastic
elastisch
élastique

715

Accent Signs

Akzentzeichen

accents

| 716a | b | c | d |

| 717a | b | c | d | e |

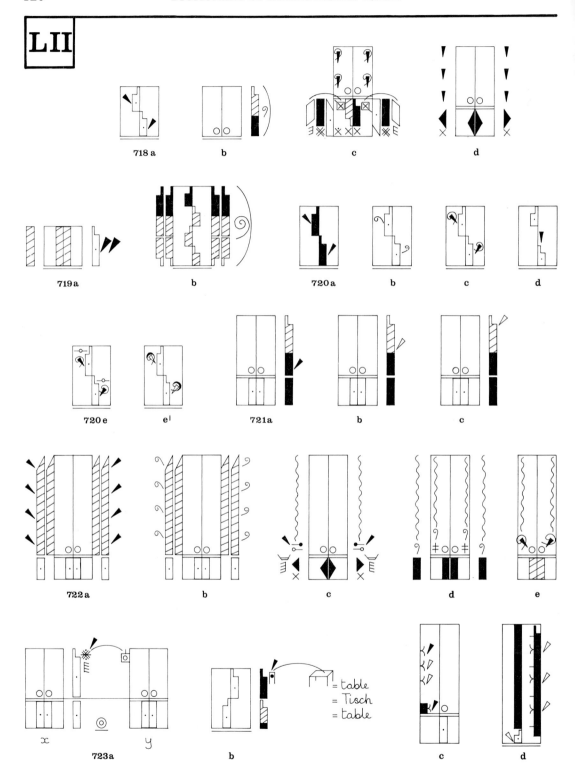

= table
= Tisch
= table

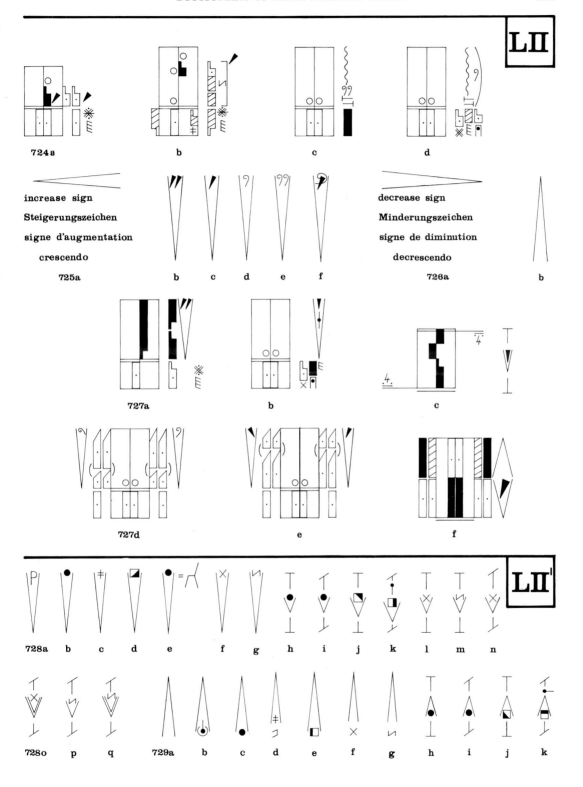

724a b c d

increase sign
Steigerungszeichen
signe d'augmentation
crescendo

725a b c d e f

decrease sign
Minderungszeichen
signe de diminution
decrescendo

726a b

727a b c

727d e f

728a b c d e f g h i j k l m n

728o p q 729a b c d e f g h i j k

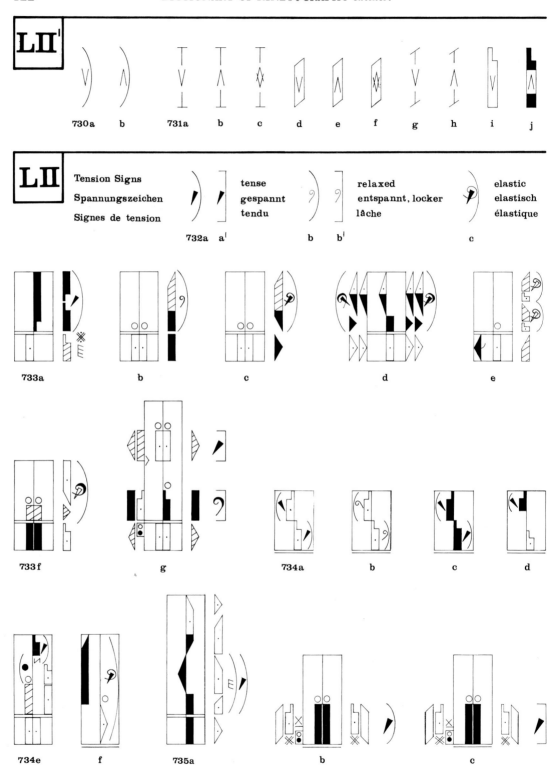

LII'

730a   b   731a   b   c   d   e   f   g   h   i   j

LII

Tension Signs		tense		relaxed		elastic
Spannungszeichen		gespannt		entspannt, locker		elastisch
Signes de tension		tendu		lâche		élastique

732a   a'   b   b'   c

733a   b   c   d   e

733f   g   734a   b   c   d

734e   f   735a   b   c

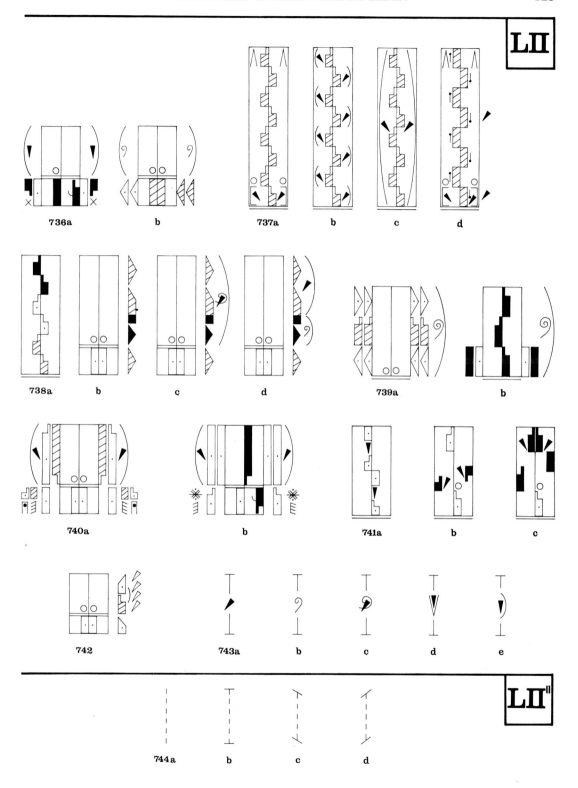

736a   b   737a   b   c   d

738a   b   c   d   739a   b

740a   b   741a   b   c

742   743a   b   c   d   e

744a   b   c   d

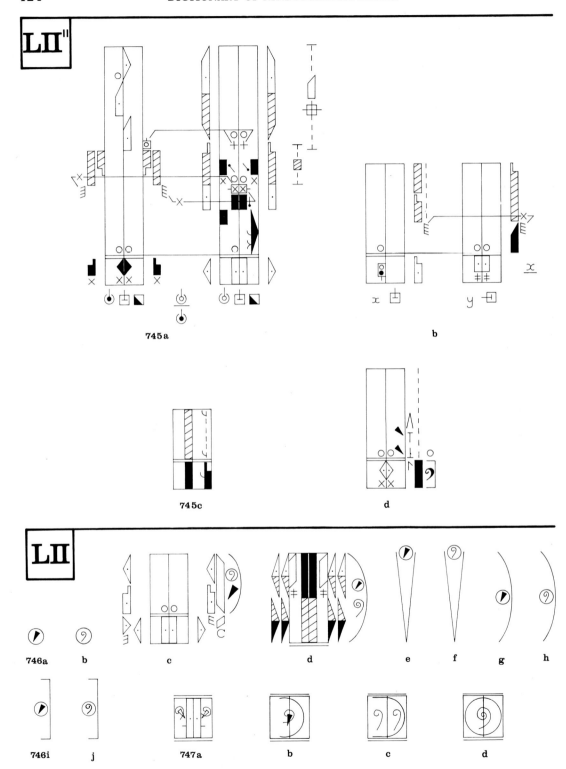

LII''

745a

b

745c

d

LII

746a   b   c   d   e   f   g   h

746i   j   747a   b   c   d

Time Measurement Signs
Die Zeitmasszeichen
Les signes de durée

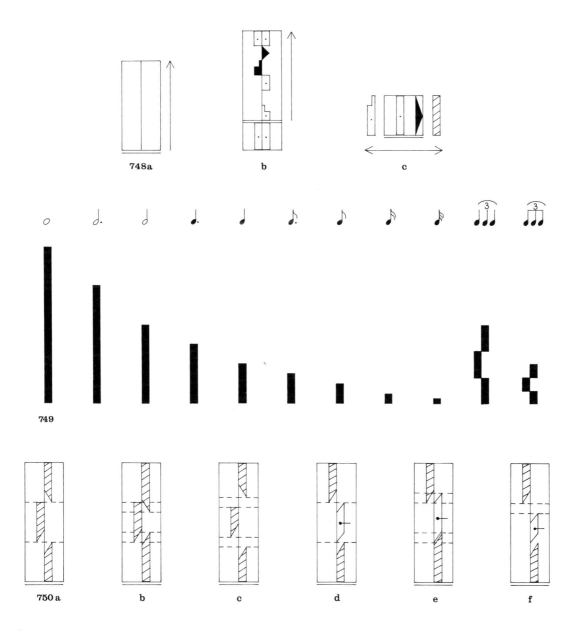

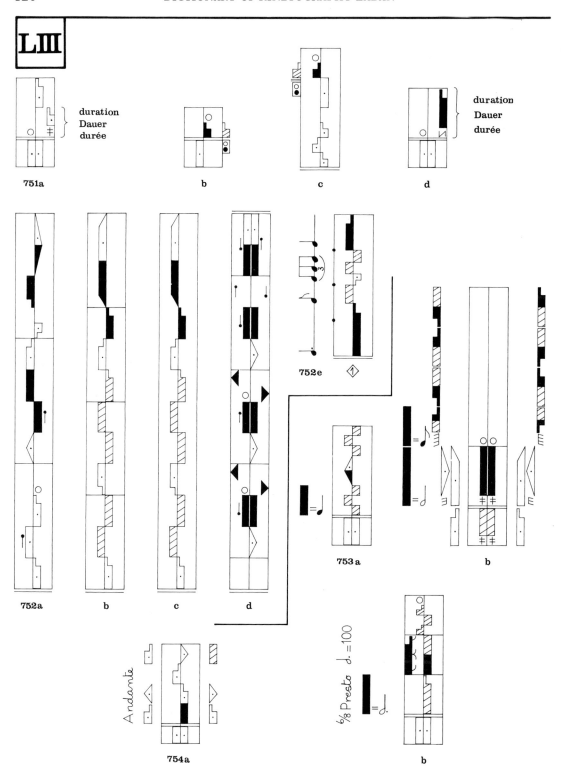

751a   duration Dauer durée

b   c   d   duration Dauer durée

752a   b   c   d

752e

753 a   b

754a   b

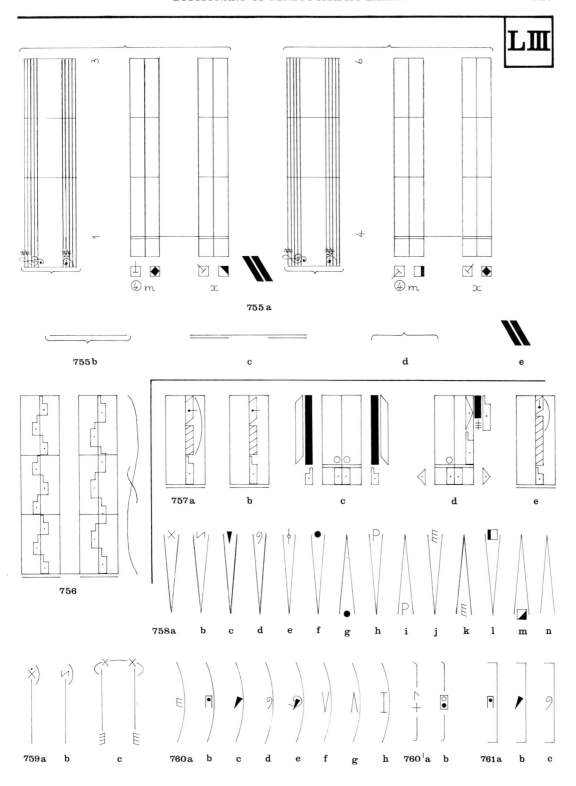

755 a

755 b   c   d   e

757 a   b   c   d   e

756

758a   b   c   d   e   f   g   h   i   j   k   l   m   n

759a   b   c   760a   b   c   d   e   f   g   h   760'a   b   761a   b   c

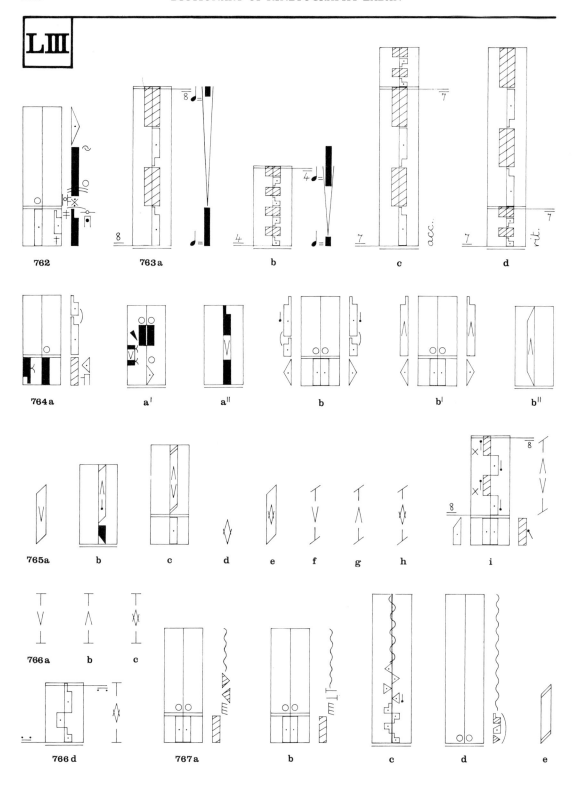

LIII

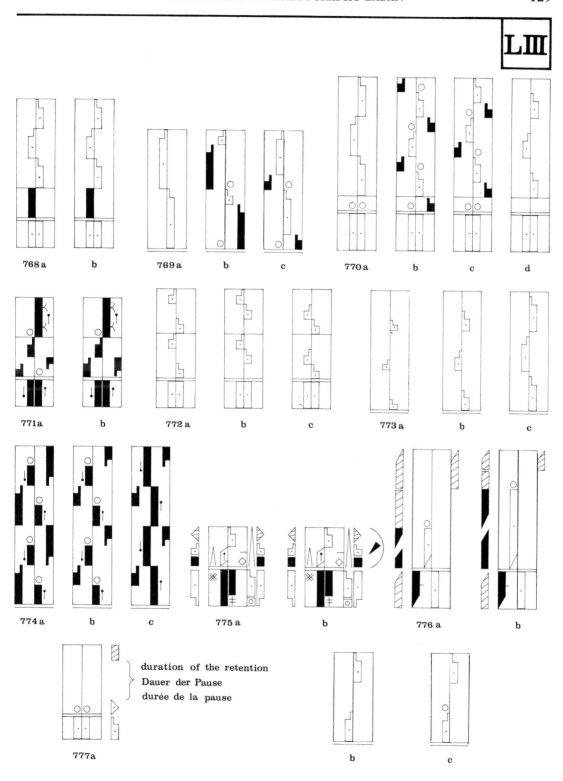

768 a   b   769 a   b   c   770 a   b   c   d

771a   b   772 a   b   c   773 a   b   c

774 a   b   c   775 a   b   776 a   b

duration of the retention
Dauer der Pause
durée de la pause

777a   b   c

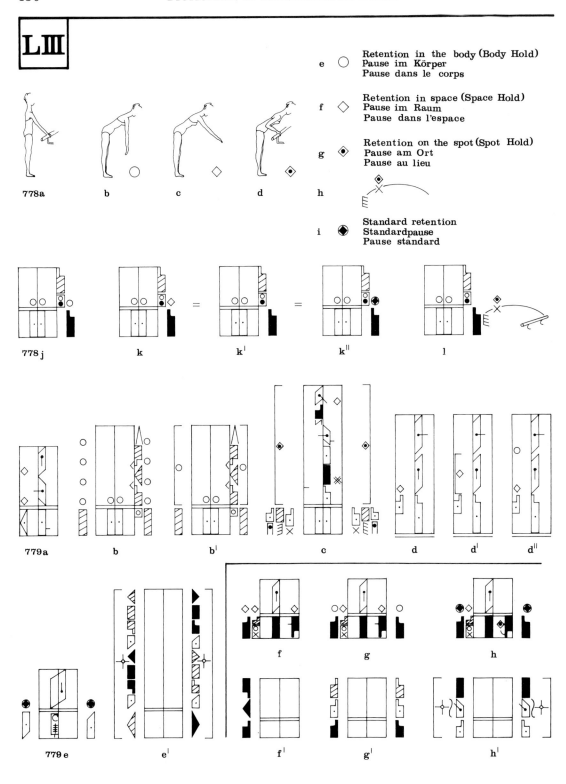

e ◯ Retention in the body (Body Hold)
    Pause im Körper
    Pause dans le corps

f ◇ Retention in space (Space Hold)
    Pause im Raum
    Pause dans l'espace

g ◈ Retention on the spot (Spot Hold)
    Pause am Ort
    Pause au lieu

h

i ◆ Standard retention
    Standardpause
    Pause standard

778a   b   c   d

778 j   k   k'   k''   l

779a   b   b'   c   d   d'   d''

779 e   e'   f'   g'   h'

f   g   h

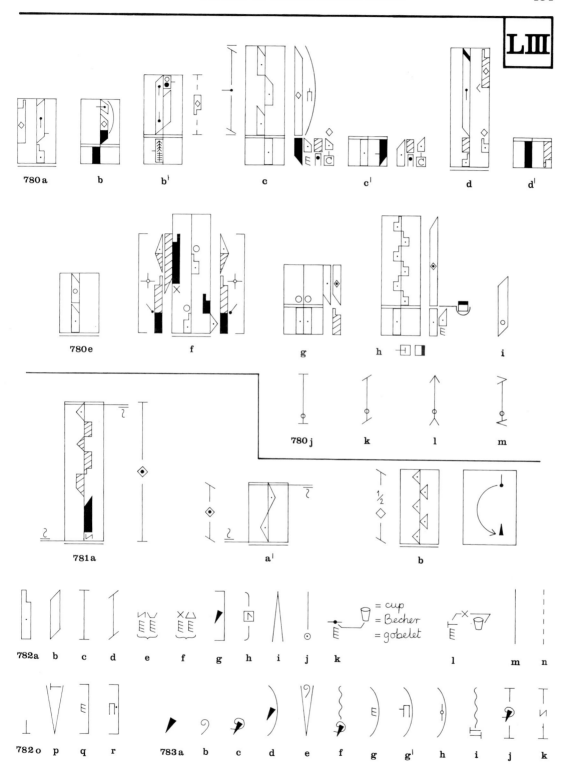

LIII

780 a   b   b¹   c   c¹   d   d¹

780 e   f   g   h   i

780 j   k   l   m

781 a   a¹   b

782 a   b   c   d   e   f   g   h   i   j   k   = cup   = Becher   = gobelet   l   m   n

782 o   p   q   r   783 a   b   c   d   e   f   g   g¹   h   i   j   k

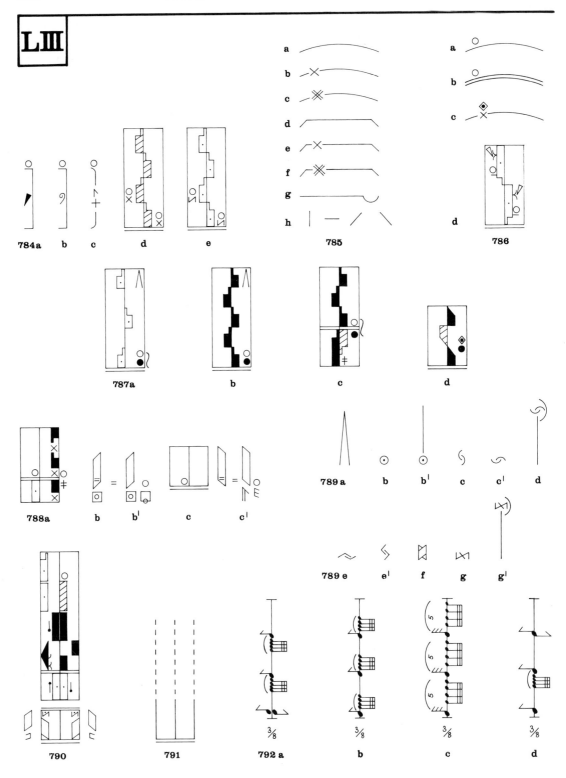

Analogy Signs
Die Entsprechungszeichen
Les signes d'analogie

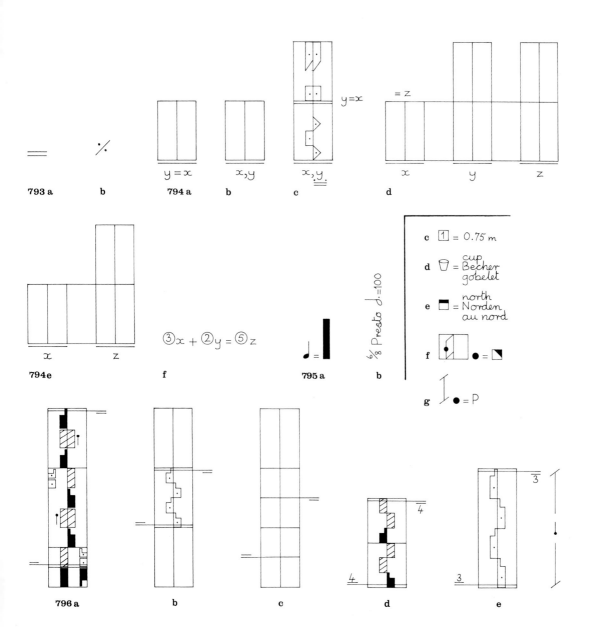

M

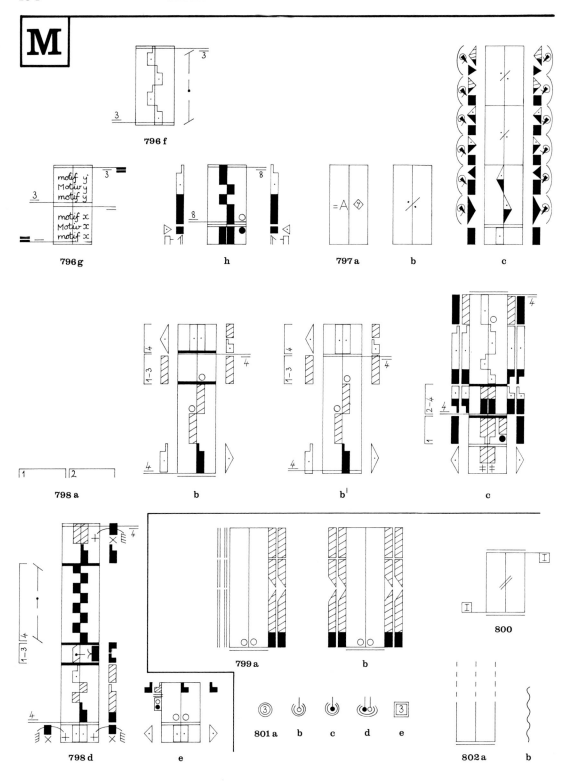

796 f

796 g   h   797 a   b   c

798 a   b   b¹   c

798 d   e   799 a   b   800

801 a   b   c   d   e   802 a   b

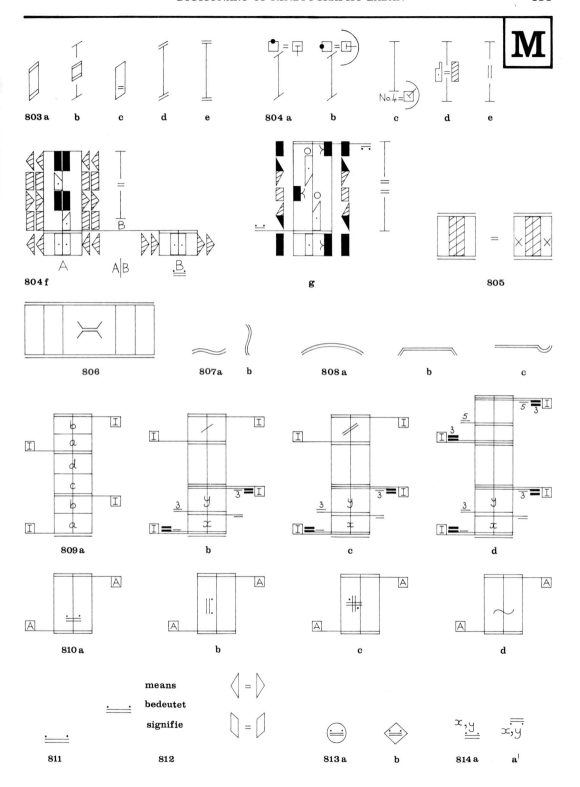

803 a   b   c   d   e   804 a   b   c   d   e

804 f   g   805

806   807 a   b   808 a   b   c

809 a   b   c   d

810 a   b   c   d

means
bedeutet
signifie

811   812   813 a   b   814 a   a'

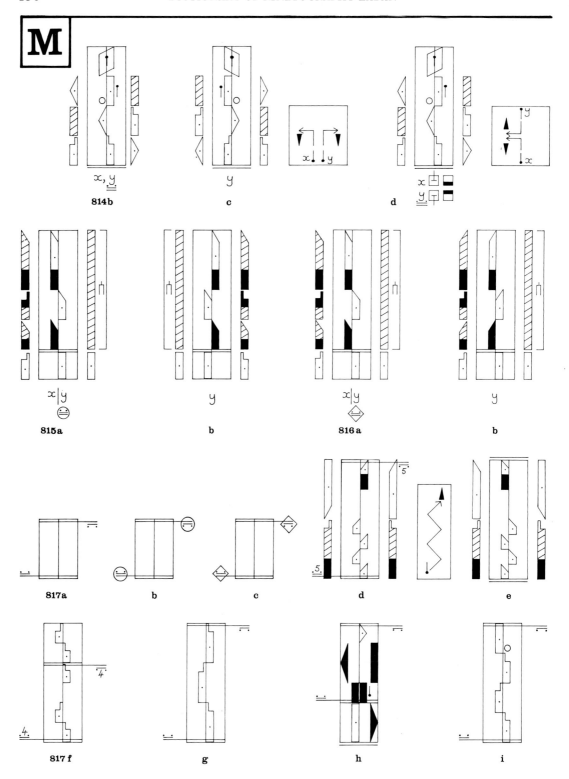

M

814b　　　　c　　　　d

x, y　　　*y*　　　*x*
　　　　　　　　　　y

815a　　　b　　　816 a　　　b

x|y　　　*y*　　　*x|y*　　　*y*

817a　　　b　　　c　　　d　　　e

817 f　　　g　　　h　　　i

M

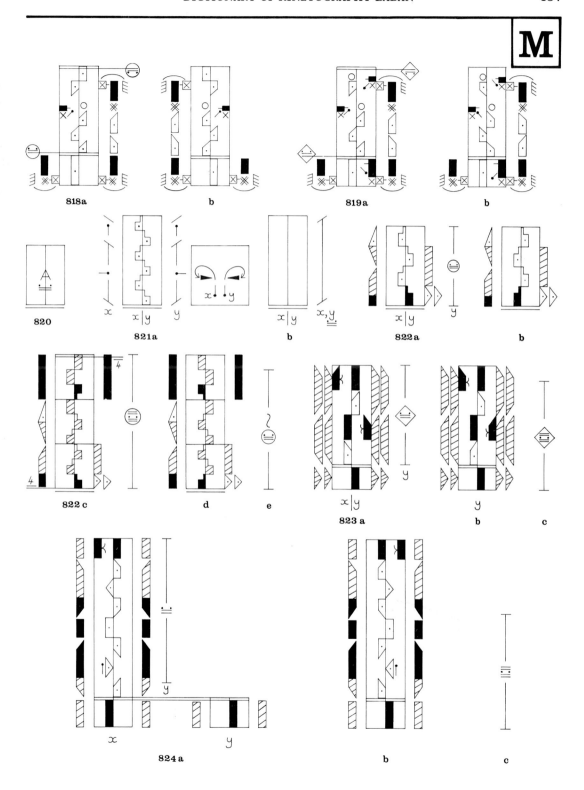

818a   b   819a   b

820   821a   b   822a   b

822 c   d   e   823 a   b   c

824 a   b   c

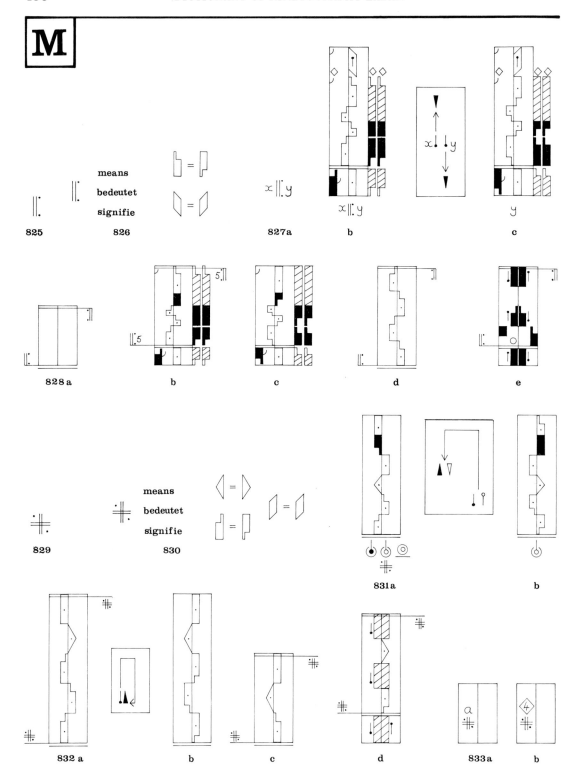

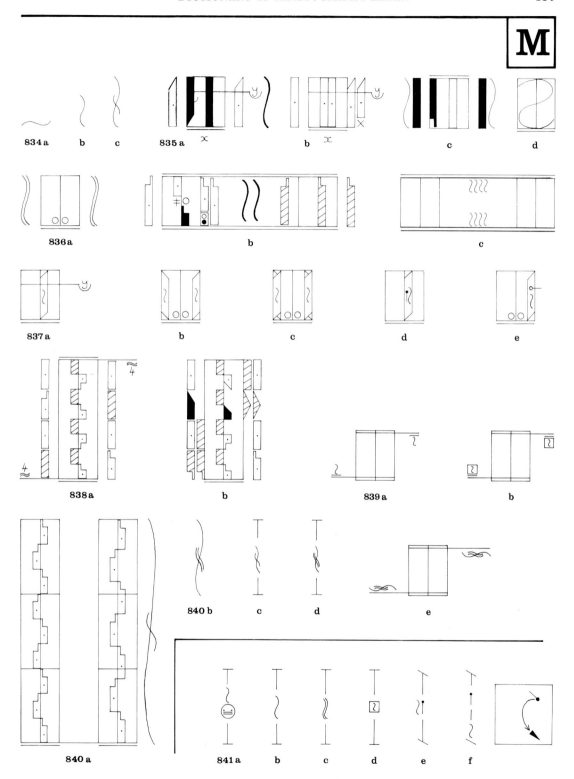

834 a   b   c   835 a   x   b   x   c   d

836 a   b   c

837 a   b   c   d   e

838 a   b   839 a   b

840 a   840 b   c   d   e

841 a   b   c   d   e   f

M

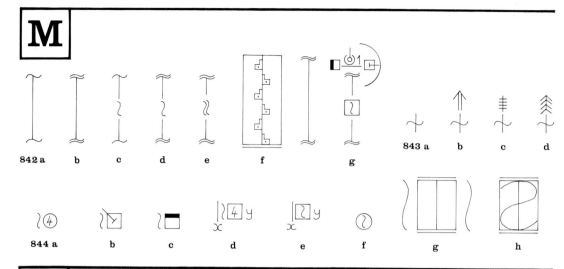

842 a   b   c   d   e   f   g   843 a   b   c   d

844 a   b   c   d   e   f   g   h

Canon Signs
Die Staffelzeichen
Les signes de canon

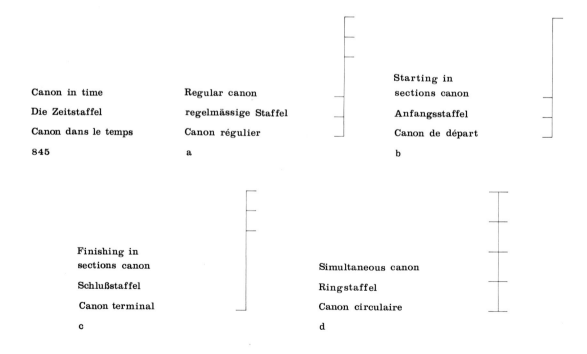

Canon in time	Regular canon	Starting in sections canon
Die Zeitstaffel	regelmässige Staffel	Anfangsstaffel
Canon dans le temps	Canon régulier	Canon de départ
845	a	b

Finishing in sections canon	Simultaneous canon
Schlußstaffel	Ringstaffel
Canon terminal	Canon circulaire
c	d

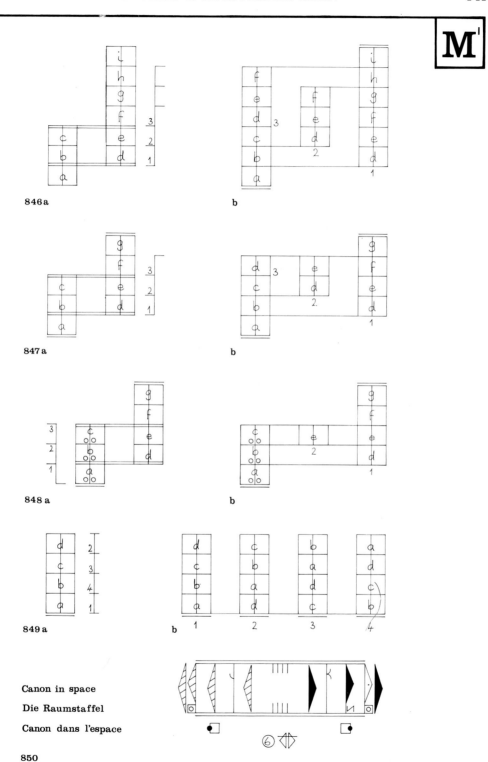

846a   b

847a   b

848a   b

849a   b

Canon in space

Die Raumstaffel

Canon dans l'espace

850

Preliminary Indications
Die Vorzeichen
Les indications préliminaires

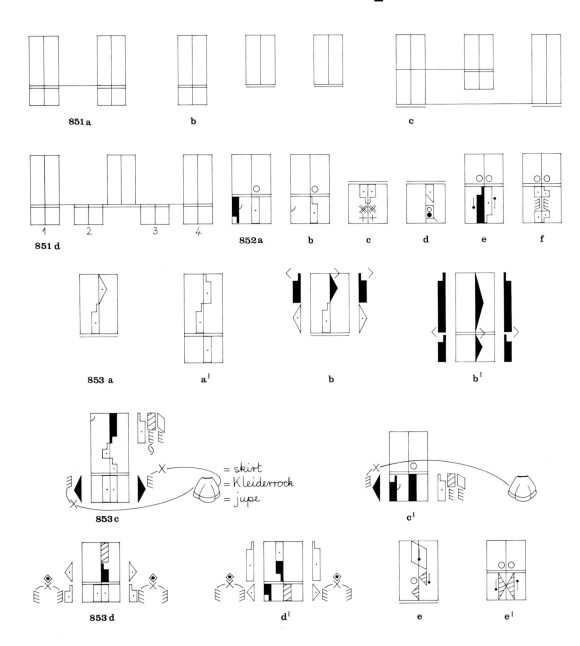

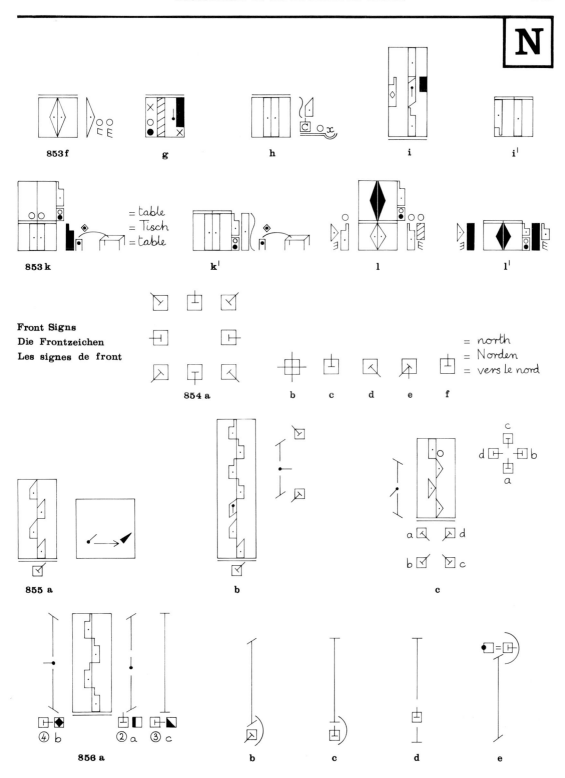

853f   g   h   i   i¹

= table
= Tisch
= table

853k   k¹   l   l¹

Front Signs
Die Frontzeichen
Les signes de front

854 a   b   c   d   e   f

= north
= Norden
= vers le nord

855 a   b   c

856 a   b   c   d   e

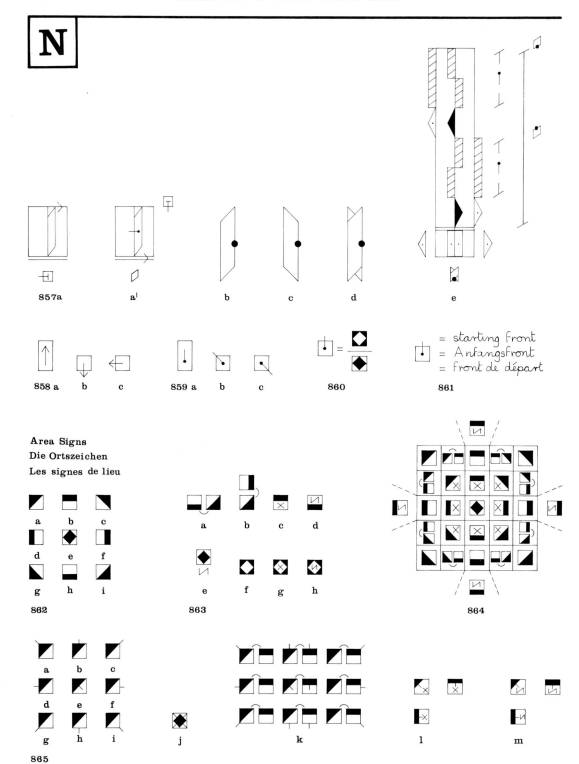

N

857a   a¹   b   c   d   e

858 a   b   c   859 a   b   c   860   861

= starting front
= Anfangsfront
= front de départ

Area Signs
Die Ortszeichen
Les signes de lieu

a   b   c
d   e   f
g   h   i

862

a   b   c   d
e   f   g   h

863

864

a   b   c
d   e   f
g   h   i   j   k   l   m

865

N

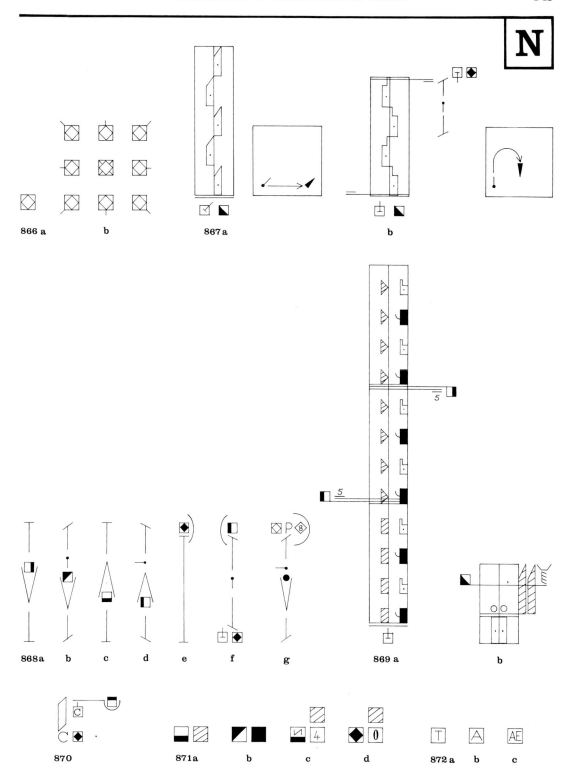

866 a   b   867 a   b

868a b c d e f g   869 a   b

870   871a b c d   872 a b c

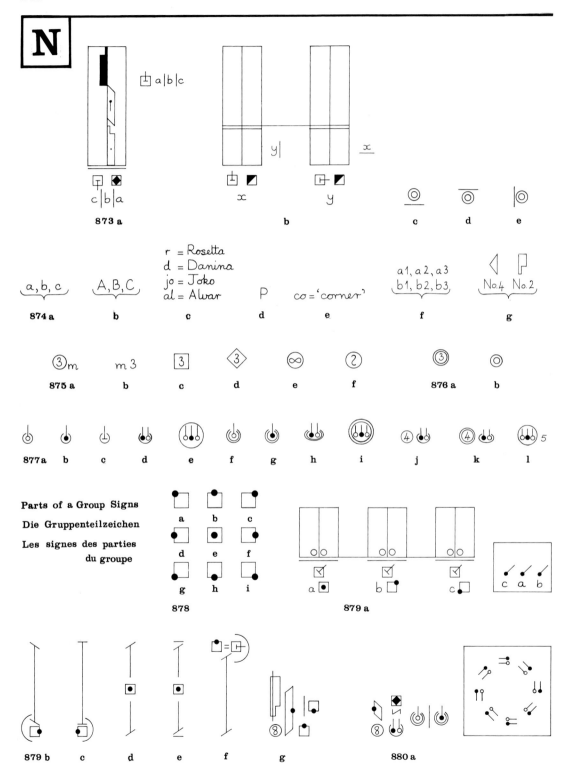

N

873 a   b   c   d   e

r = Rosetta
d = Danina
jo = Joko
al = Alvar

874 a   b   c   d   e   f   g

875 a   b   c   d   e   f   876 a   b

877 a   b   c   d   e   f   g   h   i   j   k   l

Parts of a Group Signs

Die Gruppenteilzeichen

Les signes des parties du groupe

a   b   c
d   e   f
g   h   i

878

879 a

879 b   c   d   e   f   g   880 a

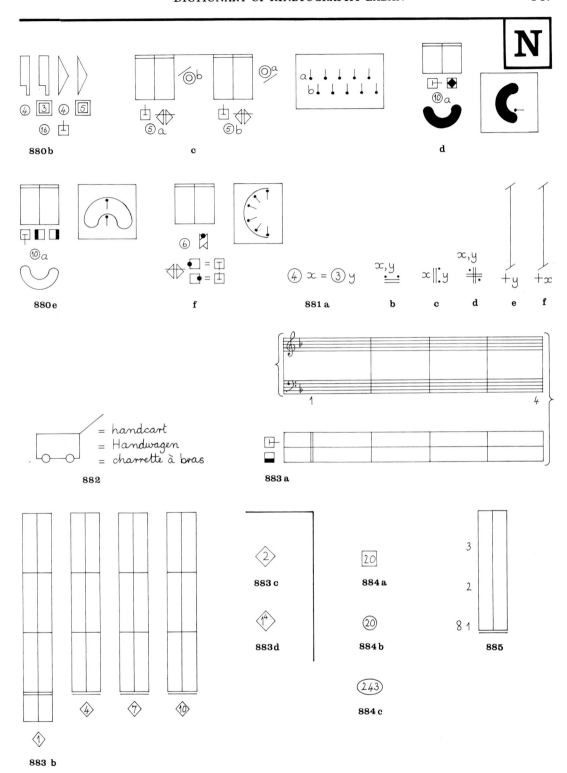

880b

c

d

880e

f

881a

b

c

d

e

f

= handcart
= Handwagen
= charrette à bras

882

883a

883c

883d

884a

884b

884c

885

883 b

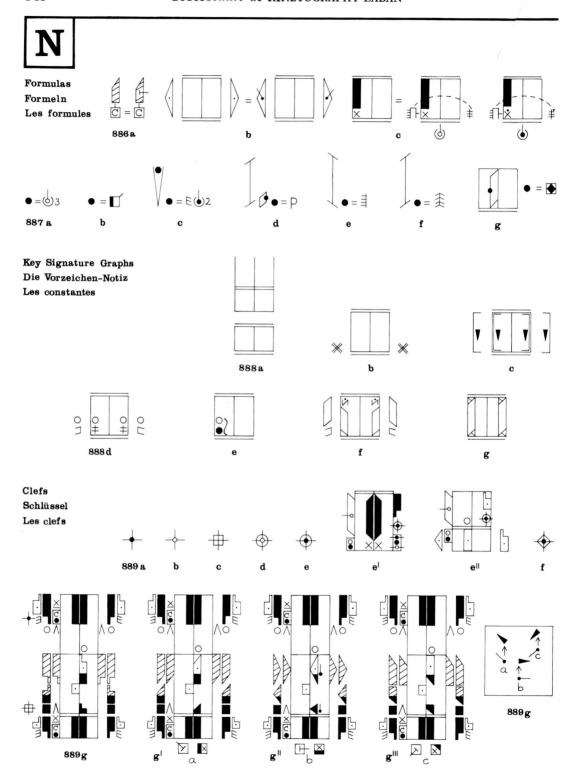

Formulas
Formeln
Les formules

886 a   b   c

887 a   b   c   d   e   f   g

Key Signature Graphs
Die Vorzeichen-Notiz
Les constantes

888 a   b   c

888 d   e   f   g

Clefs
Schlüssel
Les clefs

889 a   b   c   d   e   e^{I} e^{II} f

889 g   g^{I} a   g^{II} b   g^{III} c

889 g

N

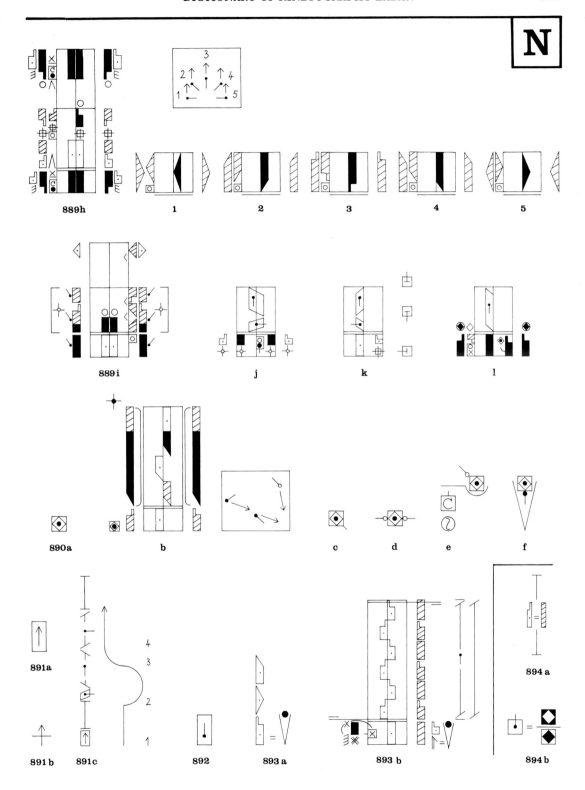

889h   1   2   3   4   5

889i   j   k   l

890a   b   c   d   e   f

891a   891b   891c   892   893a   893b   894a   894b

The Score
Die Partitur
La partition

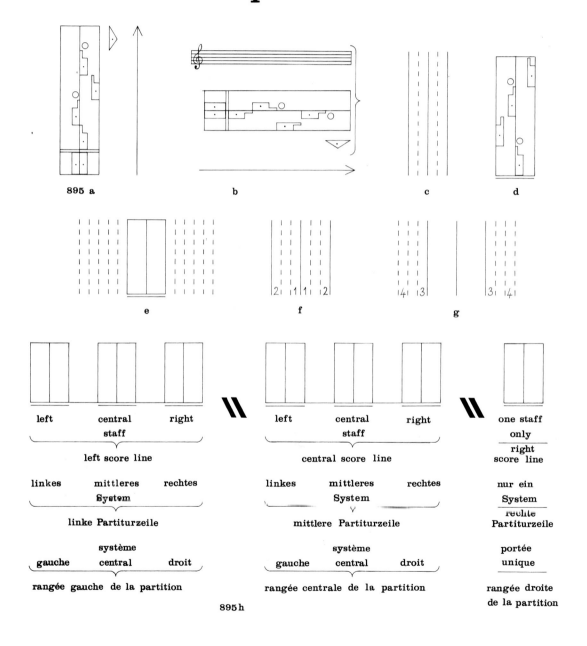

895 a   b   c   d

e   f   g

left	central staff	right		left	central staff	right		one staff only
left score line				central score line				right score line
linkes	mittleres System	rechtes		linkes	mittleres System	rechtes		nur ein System
linke Partiturzeile				mittlere Partiturzeile				rechte Partiturzeile
gauche	système central	droit		gauche	système central	droit		portée unique
rangée gauche de la partition				rangée centrale de la partition				rangée droite de la partition

895 h

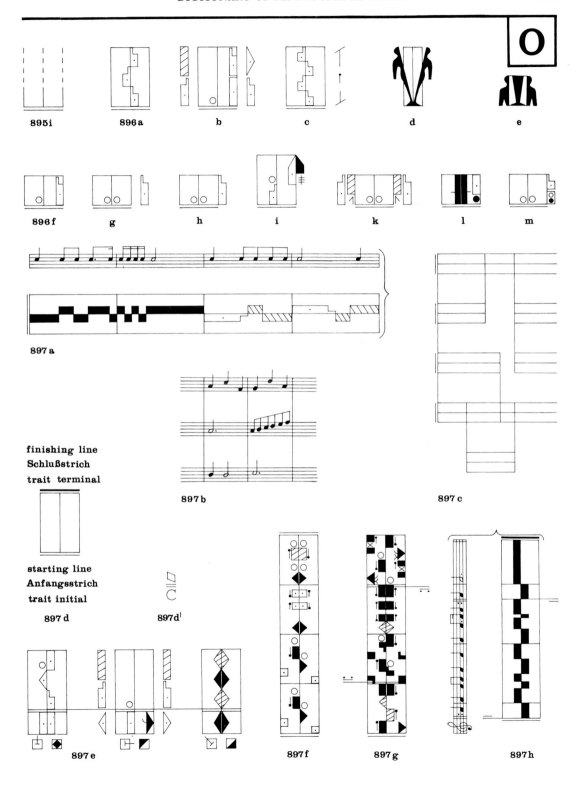

895i   896a   b   c   d   e

896f   g   h   i   k   l   m

897a

finishing line
Schlußstrich
trait terminal

897b

897c

starting line
Anfangsstrich
trait initial

897d   897d¹

897e   897f   897g   897h

O

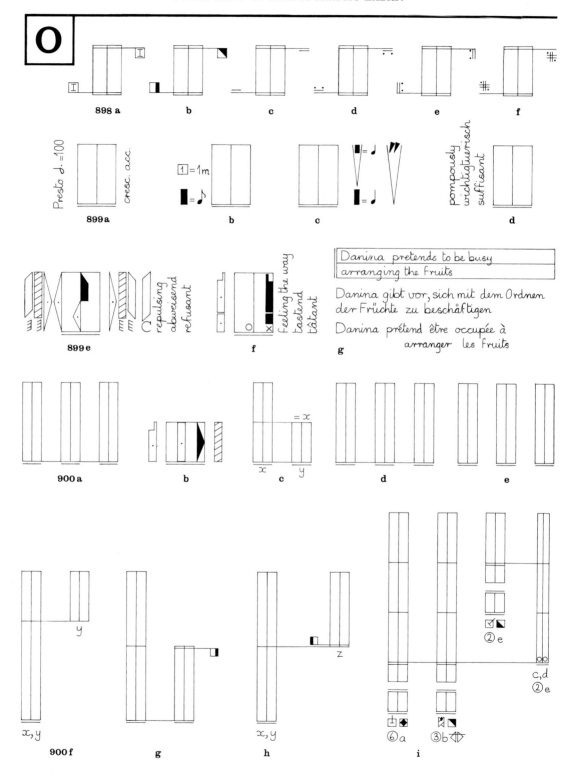

898 a   b   c   d   e   f

899 a   b   c   d

899 e   f   g

Danina pretends to be busy arranging the fruits

Danina gibt vor, sich mit dem Ordnen der Früchte zu beschäftigen

Danina prétend être occupée à arranger les fruits

900 a   b   c   d   e

900 f   g   h   i

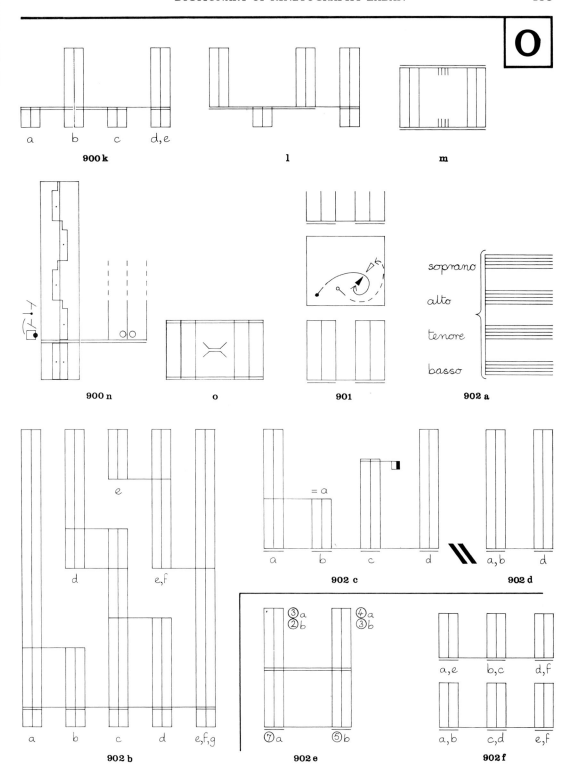

900 k   l   m

900 n   o   901   902 a

902 b

902 c   902 d

902 e   902 f

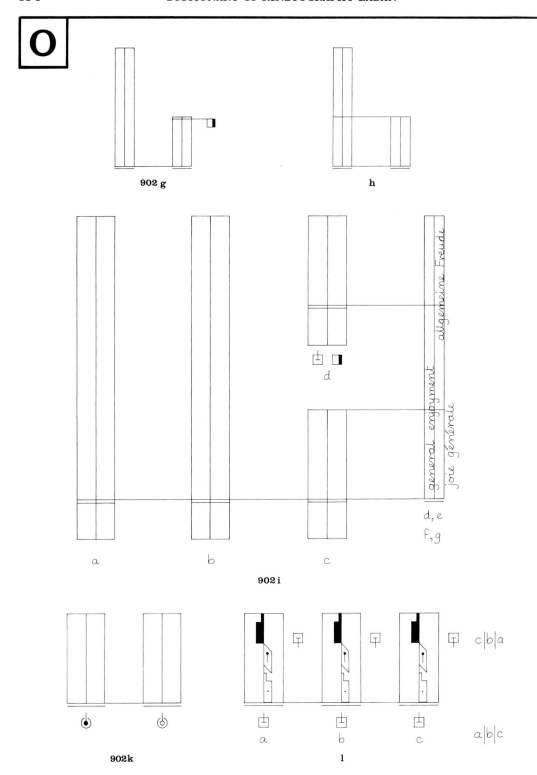

902 g   h

d

allgemeine Freude

general enjoyment

joie générale

d, e
f, g

a   b   c

902 i

c|b|a

a|b|c

902 k   l

a   b   c

Appendix I
Anhang I
Appendice I

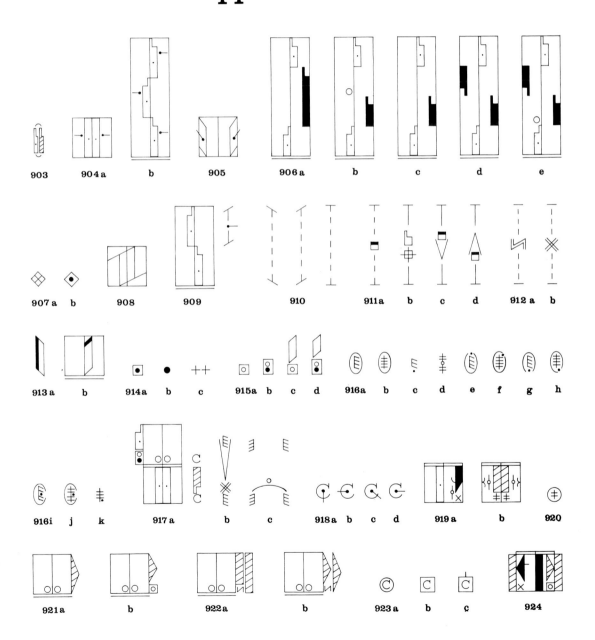

903   904 a   b   905   906 a   b   c   d   e

907 a b   908   909   910   911a b c d   912 a b

913 a b   914a b c   915a b c d   916a b c d e f g h

916i j k   917 a   b   c   918a b c d   919 a   b   920

921a   b   922a   b   923 a b c   924

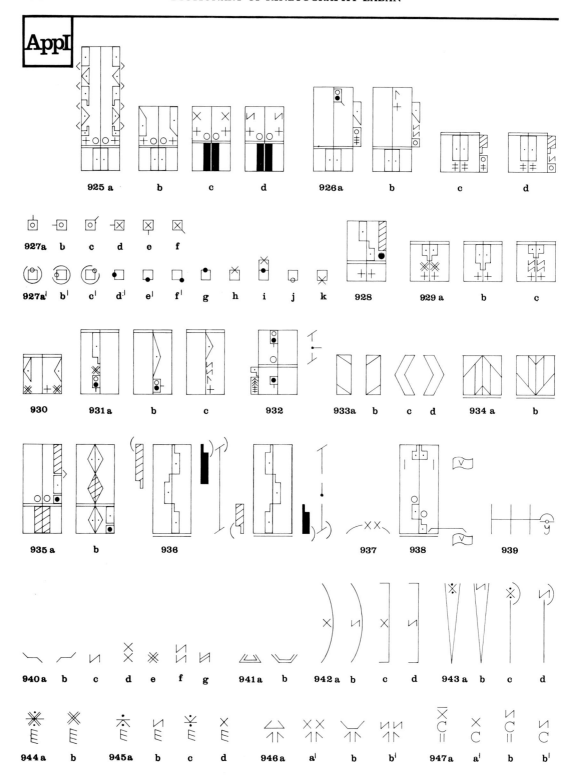

AppI

925 a   b   c   d   926a   b   c   d

927a   b   c   d   e   f

927aˡ   bˡ   cˡ   dˡ   eˡ   fˡ   g   h   i   j   k   928   929 a   b   c

930   931 a   b   c   932   933a   b   c   d   934 a   b

935 a   b   936   937   938   939

940a   b   c   d   e   f   g   941a   b   942a   b   c   d   943a   b   c   d

944 a   b   945a   b   c   d   946a   aˡ   b   bˡ   947a   aˡ   b   bˡ

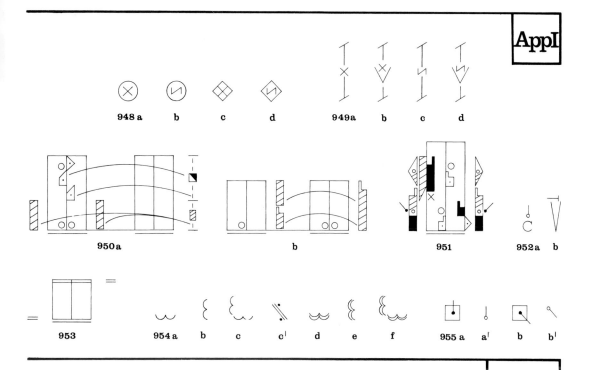

948 a   b   c   d   949a   b   c   d

950 a   b   951   952a   b

953   954 a   b   c   c'   d   e   f   955 a   a'   b   b'

Appendix II
Anhang II
Appendice II

AppII

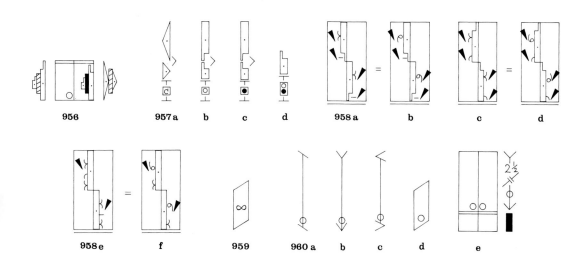

956   957a   b   c   d   958a   b   c   d

958 e   f   959   960 a   b   c   d   e

App II

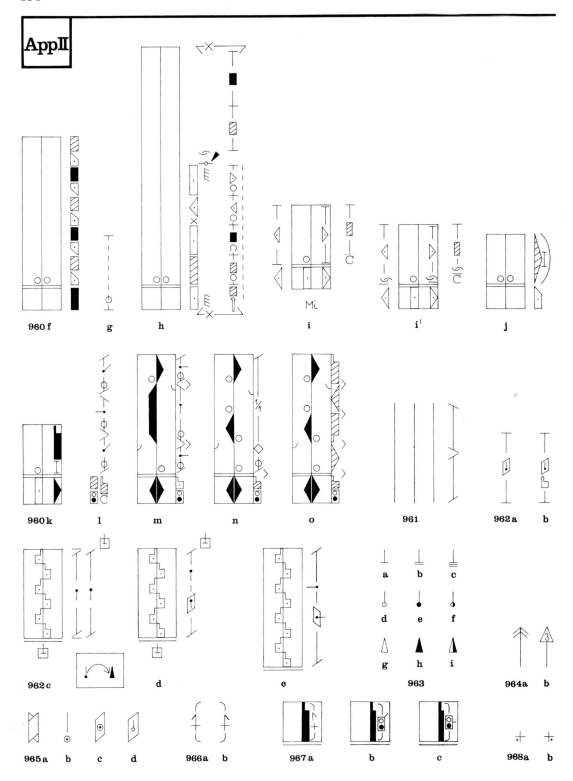

960 f   g   h   i   i¹   j

960 k   l   m   n   o   961   962 a   b

962 c   d   e   963   964 a   b

965 a   b   c   d   966 a   b   967 a   b   c   968 a   b

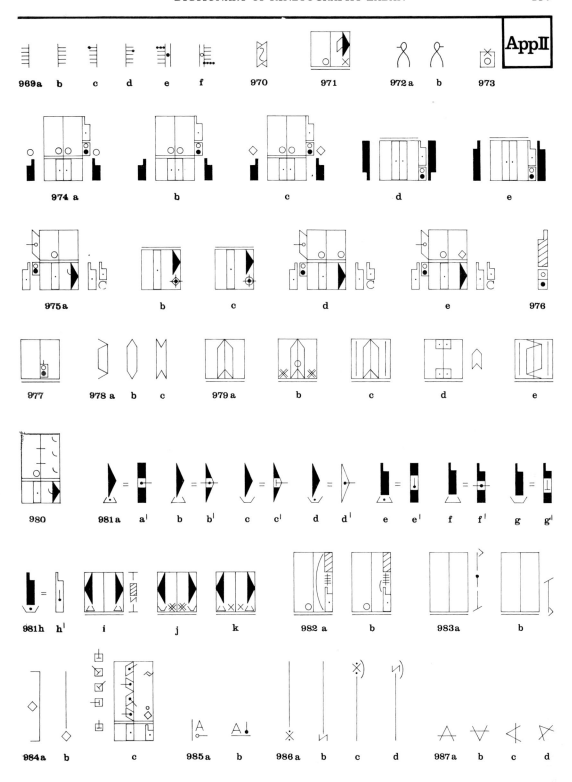

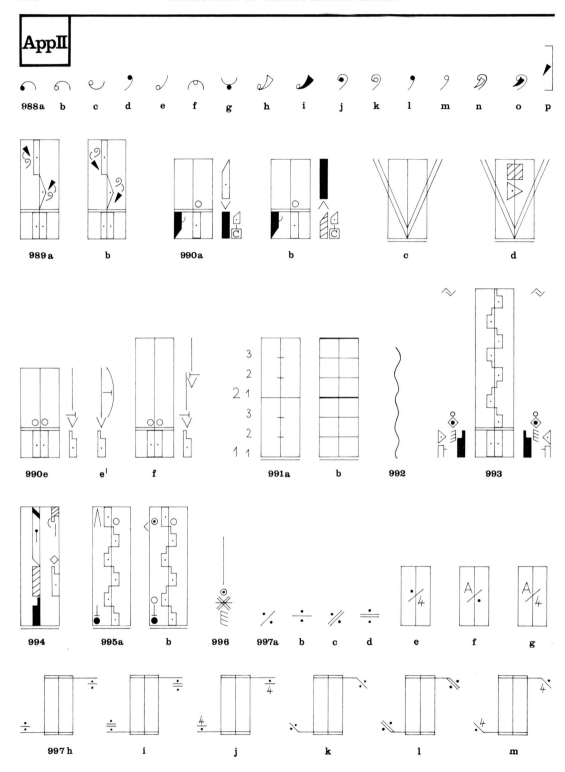

AppⅡ

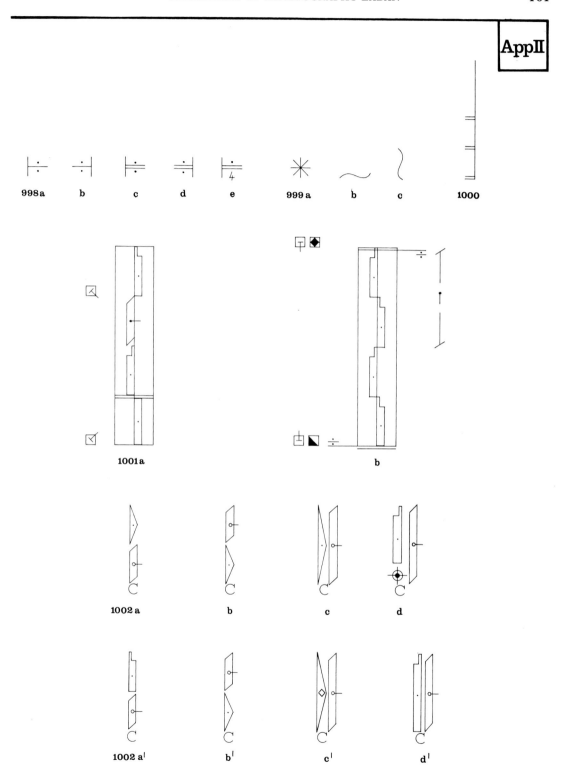

998a   b   c   d   e   999a   b   c   1000

1001a   b

1002a   b   c   d

1002a'   b'   c'   d'

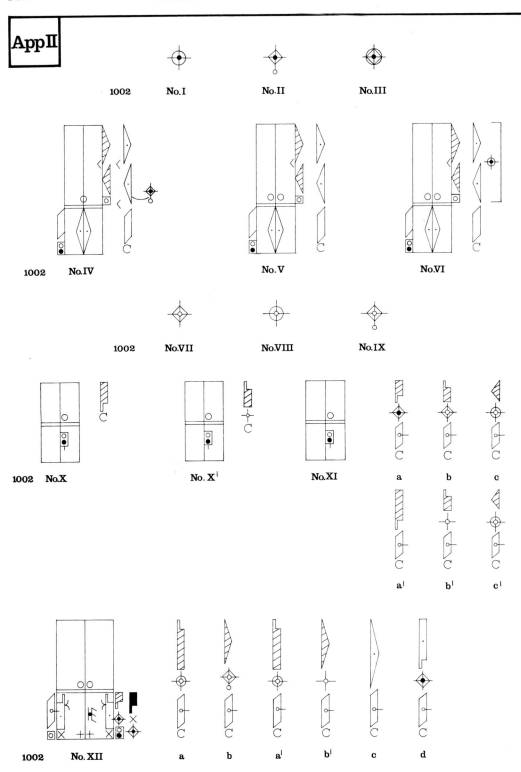